COMPLETE PREGNANCY WORKOUT GUIDE:

"Empower Your Journey to a Healthy and Fit Pregnancy"

Dr. Evelyn Stormhaven

COPYRIGHT

Contents

INTRODUCTION

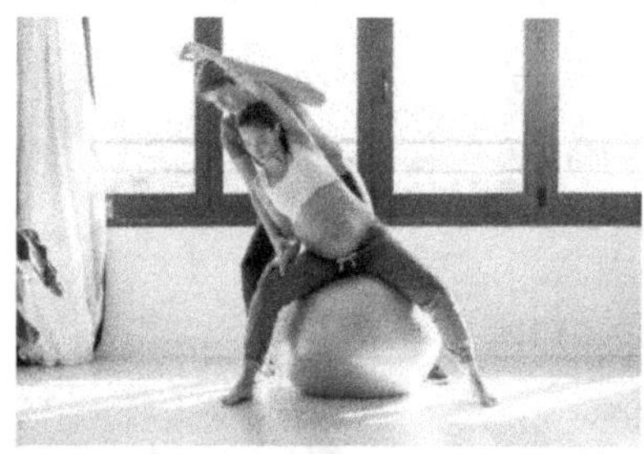 Pregnancy is a transformational and magical adventure when your body begins on an astounding voyage of change to nourish and bring forth new life. It's a phase filled with expectation, excitement and a tremendous connection to the marvel developing inside. Yet, it may also offer its fair share of discomforts and concerns, especially regarding keeping active and healthy. That's where Your Complete Pregnancy Workout Guide" comes into action as your trusty companion on this incredible adventure.

This program is not just about fitness; it's about empowerment, self-care, and recognizing the incredible strength of the female body. In the following pages, you'll find a wealth of knowledge, expert guidance, and a plan to maintain a healthy, active lifestyle throughout your pregnancy. Whether you're a fitness fanatic or someone new to exercise, "Complete Pregnancy Workout Guide" is meant to meet you where you are and help you negotiate the thrilling but often challenging pregnancy journey.

Why Exercise During Pregnancy Matters

Pregnancy brings out a torrent of changes in your body, from the fast expansion of your uterus to hormonal shifts and alterations in metabolism. These alterations might lead to pain, exhaustion, and emotional ups and downs. Exercise, however, is a vital tool that may help ease many of these symptoms, raise your energy levels, and enhance your general well-being.

As you dig into the pages of this book, you'll discover the multiple advantages of remaining active throughout pregnancy:

1. **Increased Energy:** Discover how regular physical exercise helps battle pregnant lethargy, helping you remain bright and alert.
2. **Pain Relief:** Uncover routines that address typical discomforts, including back pain, swelling ankles, and tight hips.
3. **Emotional Wellness:** Explore how exercises produce endorphins, the body's natural mood boosters, to keep you optimistic and balanced.
4. **Strengthened Core:** Learn safe and efficient ways to strengthen your core, a crucial component of a smooth pregnancy and birth.
5. **Healthy Weight Increase:** Find out how exercise may help you maintain a healthy weight increase during pregnancy.

"Complete Pregnancy Workout Guide" is not about pushing limits or establishing unrealistic objectives; it's about appreciating the beauty of exercise customized to your particular requirements and nourishing the symbiotic bond between your body and your developing baby. With advice from healthcare professionals and trained fitness experts, you can confidently begin on this path, knowing you're giving yourself and your little one the gift of health and energy.

In the following chapters, you'll discover carefully chosen exercises for each trimester, warm-up and cool-down routines, professional advice on safety considerations, and assistance in establishing a tailored training regimen. Each exercise is supported by clear directions and graphics, making it simple to follow along at your own speed and comfort level.

"Complete Pregnancy Workout Guide" is not just a book; it's a companion, a source of inspiration, and a guide to enjoying the pleasure of movement throughout pregnancy. Together, let's celebrate the extraordinary power and resilience of the female body, ensuring you begin this journey with a dazzling glow and a heart full of confidence. Welcome to "Complete Pregnancy Workout Guide."

CHAPTER ONE

The Importance of Exercise During Pregnancy

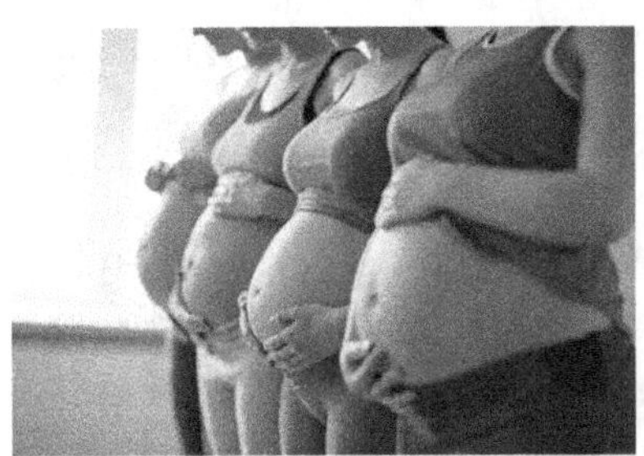

Exercise during pregnancy is of considerable relevance for the mother and the growing baby. While it's vital to contact a healthcare physician before beginning or maintaining any fitness plan during pregnancy, here are several significant reasons underscoring the value of exercise during this period:

1. **Promotes Overall Health:** Regular physical exercise may help pregnant women maintain a healthy weight, lower the risk of gestational diabetes, and enhance cardiovascular health.

2. **Enhances Mood and Reduces Stress:** Exercise causes the production of endorphins, which may help counteract mood swings, decrease stress, and create a feeling of well-being during a period when hormonal shifts can lead to emotional oscillations.

3. **Boosts Energy Levels:** Physical exercise may raise energy levels, making it easier for pregnant moms to deal

with the weariness frequently encountered throughout pregnancy.

4. **Improved Sleep:** Regular exercise may lead to healthier sleep patterns, lowering the prevalence of insomnia and helping pregnant women receive the rest they need.

5. **Prepares the Body for Labor:** Strengthening core muscles and keeping flexibility may aid with the physical demands of labor and delivery.

6. **Reduces Back discomfort:** Many pregnant women feel back discomfort as their belly develops. Properly chosen workouts may strengthen the back and abdominal muscles, thereby lowering pain.

7. **Enhances Posture:** Pregnancy may affect a woman's center of gravity, resulting in alterations in posture. Exercise may assist in improving posture and lower the chance of developing musculoskeletal disorders.

8. **Aids Digestion and Reduces Constipation:** Exercise stimulates the digestive system, helping to reduce typical pregnancy-related concerns such as constipation and bloating.

9. **Promotes Healthy Weight Gain:** Exercise may help reduce excessive weight gain during pregnancy, lowering the risk of problems including preeclampsia and gestational hypertension.

10. **Prevents Gestational Diabetes:** Regular physical exercise helps lessen the chance of developing gestational diabetes, a disease that can harm both the mother and baby's health.

11. **Boosts Circulation:** Exercise promotes blood circulation, which helps minimize the chance of developing varicose veins and swollen ankles.

12. **Fosters Healthy Fetal Development:** Research shows that maternal exercise may benefit the developing fetus, leading to enhanced fetal cardiovascular health and lower birth weight in situations of excessive mother weight gain.

13. **Eases Recovery Postpartum:** Staying active throughout pregnancy may assist in speedier postpartum recovery and help women restore their pre-pregnancy fitness levels more readily.

It's vital to realize that not all workouts are acceptable during pregnancy, and individual situations might differ. Consulting with a healthcare professional or a competent prenatal fitness specialist is vital to establishing a safe and suitable workout routine suited to the individual requirements of the pregnant woman.

Safety Precautions and Guidelines

Safety measures and recommendations are vital when it comes to exercising during pregnancy. Ensuring the well-being of both the mother and the baby is the primary concern. Here are essential safety measures and suggestions for pregnant women engaged in physical activity:

1. **Check with a Healthcare practitioner:** Before beginning or maintaining an exercise regimen during pregnancy, check with your obstetrician or healthcare practitioner. They can examine your unique health and give specific advice.

2. **Choose Safe Activities:** Opt for low-impact workouts that are less likely to produce damage or stress on the body. Examples include walking, swimming, stationary cycling, and prenatal yoga.

3. **Warm-Up and Cool-Down:** Always begin with a modest warm-up to prepare your body for activity and conclude with a cool-down to gradually drop your heart rate and avoid sudden increases in blood pressure.

4. **Stay Hydrated:** Drink lots of water before, during, and after exercise to avoid dehydration. Avoid overheating, and exercise in a well-ventilated place.

5. **Listen to Your Body:** Pay special attention to how you feel while exercising. If you feel dizziness, shortness of breath, chest discomfort, vaginal bleeding, or contractions, stop exercising immediately and seek medical assistance.

6. **Modify as Needed:**

- Adapt your workout plan as your pregnancy advances.
- Modify or remove workouts that become unpleasant or cause discomfort.
- Avoid workouts that entail resting flat on your back after the first trimester.

7. **Maintain good Form:** Use good body mechanics and form throughout activities to limit the chance of injury. Focus on calm motions and prevent overexertion.

8. **Pelvic Floor Exercises:** Include pelvic floor exercises, such as Kegels, to strengthen these muscles, which may help avoid incontinence and support the weight of your developing uterus.

9. **Avoid Overexertion:** Don't push yourself to fatigue. You should be able to carry on a conversation throughout exercising. If you can't, you may be overexerting yourself.

10. **Supportive Gear:** Wear comfortable, moisture-wicking apparel and supportive, well-fitting sports shoes that promote stability.

11. **Proper Nutrition:** Ensure you're following a balanced diet that fits your and your kid's nutritional requirements. Eat a little snack if required before exercise.

12. **Breathing methods:** Focus on suitable methods to prevent holding your breath during activity, which may contribute to higher blood pressure.

13. **Avoid High-Risk Activities:** Avoid activities with a high risk of falling, such as skiing, horseback riding, or contact sports.

14. **Posture and Alignment:** Maintain good posture and alignment during exercises to minimize the risk of back pain and strain.

15. **Regular Check-Ins:** Periodically evaluate your exercise regimen with your healthcare physician to ensure it stays safe and suitable for your changing body.

16. **Consider Prenatal Classes:** Joining prenatal fitness classes conducted by trained teachers will offer you safe and effective workout routines mainly intended for pregnancy.

Remember that every pregnancy is unique, and what is safe and pleasant for one person may not be the same for another. Always prioritize safety and speak with your healthcare practitioner for recommendations customized to your unique circumstances.

CHAPTER TWO

Planning Your Prenatal Workout Routine

Assessing Your Fitness Level

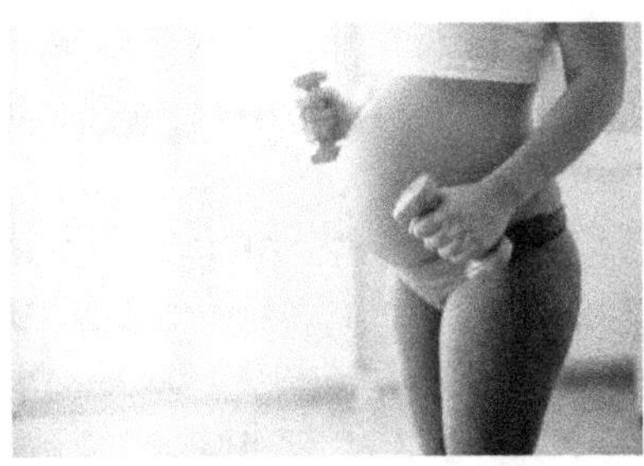

Assessing your fitness level is vital before beginning any workout program, particularly during pregnancy. It helps you identify your current physical state and personalize your exercises to your unique demands and skills. Here's how to check your fitness level while you're pregnant:

1. **Consult Your Healthcare Physician:** Before doing any fitness evaluation, consult your physician or obstetrician. They may give crucial insights into your general health and any unique issues relating to your pregnancy.

2. **Health History and Medical Evaluation:** Provide your healthcare practitioner with a comprehensive health history, including any pre-existing medical issues, prior pregnancies, or difficulties. They may undertake a medical assessment to examine your physical health and any possible risk factors.

3. **Physical Activity Questionnaire:** Fill out a physical activity questionnaire that contains data about your exercise routines, activity level, and any discomfort or pain you may be experiencing.

4. **Blood Pressure Monitoring:** Regularly monitor your blood pressure or get it tested by a healthcare expert since increased blood pressure may significantly indicate health throughout pregnancy.

5. **Heart Rate Monitoring:** During activity, monitor your heart rate. You may use a heart rate monitor or measure your pulse manually. Ensure that your heart rate stays within the safe range your healthcare expert indicates.

6. **Body Composition:** Assess your body composition to establish your body fat percentage. You may employ procedures like skinfold calipers, bioelectrical impedance scales, or expert body composition examinations.

7. **Strength and Flexibility Testing:** Evaluate your strength and flexibility, considering that pregnant hormones may impact your joint flexibility. Simple tests like leg lifts, squats, and light stretching may give information.

8. **Balance and Coordination:** Pay attention to your balance and coordination since they may vary throughout pregnancy owing to adjustments in your center of gravity.

You may undertake balancing exercises, such as standing on one leg, with support nearby for safety.

9. **Functional Fitness Assessment:** Assess your capacity to execute everyday tasks, such as getting up from a chair, ascending stairs, and lifting light things. This can help you discover any areas of weakness or pain.

10. **Listen to Your Body:** During self-assessment or exercises, listen to your body. If you develop pain, discomfort, dizziness, or shortness of breath, discontinue the activity immediately and talk with your healthcare professional.

11. **Keep a Fitness notebook:** Maintain a fitness notebook to monitor your exercises, how you feel during and after exercise, and any changes in your physical condition. This may help you track progress and make required modifications.

12. **Develop realistic objectives:** Based on your fitness evaluation and in cooperation with your healthcare practitioner, develop realistic fitness objectives for your pregnancy. These objectives should be explicit, quantifiable, and customized to your requirements and constraints.

Remember that pregnancy is a unique experience for each woman, and your fitness level and demands may alter throughout. Regular contact with your healthcare practitioner is crucial to ensure your exercise program is safe and helpful for you and your developing baby. Adjust your exercises to meet your changing body and keep in sync with your physical state throughout your pregnancy.

Setting Realistic Goals

Setting realistic fitness goals throughout pregnancy is vital to maintain a safe and successful training regimen that matches your changing body and requirements. Here are some recommendations on how to make realistic exercise goals during pregnancy:

1. **Consult with Your Healthcare Provider:** Discuss your fitness objectives with your physician or obstetrician. They may give advice based on your medical history, present health, and any unique issues connected to your pregnancy.

2. **Consider Your Pre-Pregnancy Fitness Level:** Consider your fitness level before pregnancy. If you were previously active, you may have different objectives than someone less active.

3. **Be Realistic About Changes:** Understand that your body is experiencing significant changes, and your workout program must adjust appropriately. Set feasible objectives considering your present physical state and the limits imposed by pregnancy.

4. **Focus on Maintenance:** For many pregnant women, maintaining their fitness level is feasible. This implies regularly exercising to keep strength, flexibility, and cardiovascular fitness rather than seeking dramatic increases.

5. **Prioritize Safety:** Safety should be the top focus. Your objectives should promote the well-being of both you and your kid. Avoid high-risk or vigorous activities that might harm your pregnancy.

6. **Set Specific and quantifiable objectives:** Clearly describe and make your objectives quantifiable. For example, instead of a generic aim like "stay active," make a precise objective like "engage in 30 minutes of moderate-intensity exercise at least four times a week."

7. **Gradual Progression:** If you aim to enhance your fitness level, do it gradually. Focus on small progress and avoid pushing yourself too much. Remember that pregnancy is not the time for strenuous exercise regimes.

8. **Account for Weariness and Discomfort:** Recognize that pregnant weariness and discomfort might limit your workout ability. Adjust your objectives as required to suit these circumstances.

9. **Include Non-Fitness objectives:** Consider defining objectives linked to general health and well-being. This

might include objectives relating to diet, stress management, and obtaining appropriate rest.

10. **Stay Flexible:** Be prepared to change your objectives as your pregnancy advances. Your body will change, and your workout choices and skills may evolve.

11. **Seek advice:** Enlist the advice of a trained pregnant fitness professional or attend prenatal exercise programs where you may receive guidance on developing and attaining safe and realistic fitness goals.

12. **Celebrate Achievements:** Celebrate your successes, no matter how modest they appear. Whether finishing a workout or just keeping active, each victory is a step toward more excellent health for you and your kid.

Remember that every pregnancy is unique, and what is reasonable for one person may not be the same for another. The idea is to communicate openly with your healthcare practitioner, listen to your body, and change your objectives and exercise program to promote a healthy and safe pregnancy. Prioritizing your well-being and your kid's is the ultimate objective during this unique time.

Choosing the Right Exercises

Selecting the correct workouts during pregnancy is vital for safeguarding both your safety and the well-being of your growing baby. Here are recommendations for selecting the correct workouts during pregnancy:

1. **Consult with Your Healthcare Practitioner:** Always consult your healthcare practitioner or obstetrician before beginning any workout regimen during pregnancy. They may make individualized suggestions based on your medical history and current condition.

2. **Low-Impact Activities:** Focus on low-impact activities that are easy on your joints and limit the chance of damage. Examples include walking, swimming, stationary cycling, and water aerobics.

3. **Prenatal Fitness Classes:** Consider taking prenatal fitness classes or hiring a professional prenatal fitness teacher. These sessions are created exclusively for pregnant women and deliver safe and efficient exercises.

4. **Aerobic Exercise:** Aerobic or cardiovascular workouts assist in preserving fitness and stamina. Opt for moderate-intensity exercises that enable you to hold a conversation while exercising. Good alternatives include brisk walking, low-impact aerobics, and dance.

5. **Strength Training:** Strength training may assist in maintaining muscular tone and prepare your body for the physical demands of work. Use low to moderate weights and concentrate on controlled full-range motions. Avoid

heavy lifting and workouts that strain the abdominal muscles.

6. **Flexibility & Stretching:** Stretching exercises may increase flexibility and minimize the risk of muscular stress and cramping. Incorporate mild stretching regimens, including yoga and pregnant Pilates.

7. **Pelvic Floor Exercises:** Pelvic floor exercises, such as Kegels, are vital for maintaining pelvic health and may help avoid incontinence difficulties throughout pregnancy and postpartum.

8. **Balance and Stability:** Balance and stability exercises may improve coordination and lessen the chance of falls, particularly when your center of gravity moves. Include exercises like single-leg balancing and stability ball exercises with sufficient support.

9. **Breathing methods:** Learn and practice correct breathing methods to increase relaxation and manage stress. Controlled breathing may also be advantageous during childbirth.

10. **Avoid High-Risk Activities:** Avoid activities with a high risk of falling or injury, such as contact sports, horseback riding, skiing, and activities that entail quick changes in direction.

11. **Listen to Your Body:** Pay careful attention to your body's cues throughout the activity. If you develop pain, dizziness, shortness of breath, or other discomfort, discontinue the exercise immediately and talk with your healthcare professional.

12. **Change as Needed:** As your pregnancy continues, you may need to change workouts or adopt other more pleasant motions. For example, you may need to move from high-impact aerobics to low-impact or swimming.

13. **Stay Hydrated:** Drink lots of water before, during, and after exercise to avoid dehydration. Avoid overheating, and exercise in a well-ventilated setting.

14. **Wear Comfortable Clothing:** Choose moisture-wicking and breathable clothing that fits comfortably to suit your changing physique. Supportive footwear is also necessary.

15. **Posture and Alignment:** Maintain appropriate posture and alignment throughout activities to limit the risk of back discomfort and strain. Avoid resting flat on your back after the first trimester.

16. **Range and Enjoyment:** Keep your workouts fun by including a range of routines. This may help you remain motivated and involved throughout your pregnancy.

Remember that every pregnancy is different, and individual circumstances vary. What's most essential is that you pick activities that correlate with your fitness level, comfort, and health state and that you do so under the advice of your healthcare practitioner. Prioritizing safety and well-being is crucial throughout pregnancy.

Creating a Weekly Workout Schedule

Creating a weekly fitness regimen during pregnancy requires careful preparation to maintain a safe and effective exercise routine while considering your changing body and energy levels. Here's a step-by-step approach to help you construct a proper weekly fitness schedule:

Step 1: Consult with Your Healthcare Provider

Before creating your fitness routine, talk with your healthcare physician or obstetrician. Discuss any medical issues in your fitness objectives, and receive approval to exercise throughout pregnancy.

Step 2: Determine Your Available Time

Consider your daily and weekly obligations, including job, family, and other duties. Determine how much time you can commit to working out each day.

Step 3: Choose Your Exercise Activities

Pick acceptable fitness activities for your pregnancy based on your healthcare provider's suggestions and preferences. This may involve aerobic, weight training, flexibility, and balancing activities.

Step 4: Set Weekly Exercise Goals

Establish defined, quantifiable, and attainable workout objectives. Consider both short-term and long-term aims. For example, your objective may be to accomplish 150 minutes of moderate-intensity aerobic activity per week.

Step 5: Divide Your Workout Routine

Divide your preferred workouts into categories, such as aerobic, strength, flexibility, and balance. Determine how many days per week you'll interact in each area.

Step 6: Incorporate Rest Days

Schedule rest days to enable your body to recuperate and avoid the danger of overexertion. Rest is crucial throughout pregnancy, so schedule at least one or two weekly rest days.

Step 7: Consider Trimester-Specific Needs

Recognize that your workout program may need to adjust as your pregnancy advances. Tailor your routines to meet each trimester's physical changes and discomforts.

Sample Weekly Workout Schedule

Here's an example of a weekly fitness routine for a pregnant lady. Remember that this is a basic guideline, and individual requirements may vary:

Trimester 1 (Weeks 1-12):
- **Monday:** 30 minutes of prenatal yoga or light stretching
- **Tuesday:** 20-30 minutes of low-impact aerobic activity (e.g., brisk walking)
- **Wednesday:** Rest or light, leisurely activity (e.g., swimming)
- **Thursday:** 20-30 minutes of strength training with light weights
- **Friday:** 20-30 minutes of prenatal Pilates
- **Saturday:** Rest or mild yoga
- **Sunday:** 20-30 minutes of low-impact aerobic exercise. Trimester 2 (Weeks 13-27):

- **Monday:** 30-40 minutes of prenatal yoga or light stretching
- **Tuesday:** 20-30 minutes of low-impact aerobic exercise
- **Wednesday:** 20-30 minutes of strength training with mild to moderate weights
- **Thursday:** 20-30 minutes of prenatal Pilates
- **Friday:** Rest or mild, relaxed activities
- **Saturday:** 20-30 minutes of low-impact aerobic exercise
- **Sunday:** Rest or mild yoga Trimester 3 (Weeks 28-40):

- **Monday:** 30-40 minutes of prenatal yoga or light stretching
- **Tuesday:** 20-30 minutes of low-impact aerobic exercise
- **Wednesday:** 20-30 minutes of strength training with light weights
- **Thursday:** 20-30 minutes of prenatal Pilates
- **Friday:** Rest or mild, relaxed activities
- **Saturday:** 20-30 minutes of low-impact aerobic exercise
- **Sunday:** Rest or mild yoga

Remember to alter your schedule as required, listen to your body, and check your healthcare practitioner often to ensure your exercise program stays safe and suitable for your pregnancy. Prioritize flexibility and be open to altering your schedule depending on how you feel each day.

CHAPTER THREE

Warm-up and Cool-down

Warm-Up Exercises

Neck Rolls

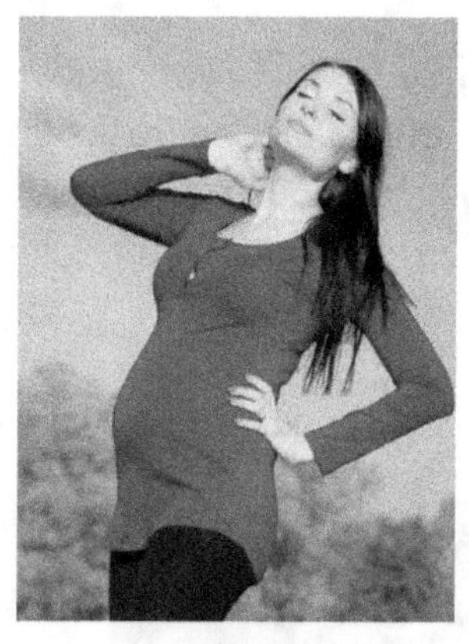

Neck rolls are a simple and efficient stretching exercise that may help reduce tension in the neck and shoulders, which is particularly good for pregnant women who may feel higher stress in these regions owing to changes in posture and weight distribution. Here's how to execute neck rolls safely during pregnancy:

Instructions:

1. **Sit or Stand Tall:** Find a comfortable and sturdy sitting or standing posture. Ensure that your feet are hip-width apart if you're standing and your back is well-supported if you're seated.

2. **Relax Your Shoulders:** Begin with relaxed shoulders, away from your ears.

3. **Chin to Chest:** Gently drop your chin towards your chest. Go as far as is comfortable, and avoid pushing your head down.

4. **Move to the Right:** Slowly move your head to the right, putting your right ear towards your right shoulder. Keep the movement slow and controlled.

5. **Hold for a Breath:** Pause for a breath or two in this posture, feeling the stretch down the left side of your neck.

6. **Roll to the Back:** Continue the circular motion by leaning your head backward softly. Avoid leaning your head too far back, particularly during the latter stages of pregnancy when equilibrium might be impaired.

7. **Roll to the Left:** Complete the circle by bringing your left ear towards your left shoulder. Again, hold for a breath or two, feeling the stretch down the right side of your neck.

8. **Repeat in the Opposite Direction:** If you like, you may reverse the direction of the neck roll by beginning with your left ear towards your left shoulder and then rolling your head to the rear, right ear to the right shoulder, and back to the front.

9. **Repeat Several Times:** Continue moving your neck gently in one way and then the other for around 30

seconds to 1 minute, or as long as it feels comfortable and calming.

10. **Maintain a calm Pace:** Ensure the motions are calm and controlled, and never push your neck into any position that feels unpleasant or causes discomfort.

11. **Finish with a Neutral posture:** After completing the neck rolls, bring your head to a neutral, upright posture, and take a minute to relax your shoulders.

Neck rolls are a terrific technique to reduce neck and shoulder strain, enhance circulation in the region, and promote relaxation. However, be careful of any pain or dizziness during pregnancy, and if you encounter any alarming symptoms, cease the activity immediately. If you have any concerns or underlying medical issues, see your healthcare professional before beginning or maintaining any fitness regimen during pregnancy.

Shoulder Shrugs

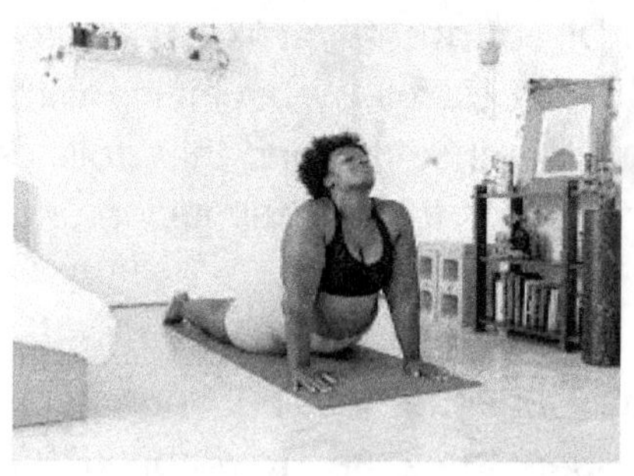

Shoulder shrugs are a simple but effective exercise to help reduce stress and pain in the shoulder and neck region. They may be especially effective for pregnant women who may feel higher tension and muscular stiffness in these regions owing to changes in posture and weight distribution. Here's how to execute shoulder shrugs safely during pregnancy:

Instructions:
1. **Stand or Sit Comfortably:** Find a comfortable and stable sitting or standing posture. Ensure that your feet are hip-width apart if you're standing and your back is well-supported if you're seated.

2. **Relax Your Arms:** Let your arms hang naturally at your sides, and keep your hands relaxed.

3. **Engage Your Core:** Gently engage your abdominal muscles to support your lower back and maintain excellent posture.

4. **Shrug Your Shoulders:** Inhale deeply and, as you exhale, gently pull both shoulders up toward your ears in a calm, controlled motion. Imagine attempting to connect your shoulders to your ears.

5. **Hold for a period:** Hold your shoulders in the shrugging posture for a little to feel the stretch and tension dissipate in your neck and upper back.

6. **Relax and drop:** As you inhale, softly drop your shoulders back to their natural posture. Imagine getting rid of any tension or stress in this movement.

7. **Repeat Several Times:** Perform the shoulder shrug exercise for roughly 10-15 repetitions, or as long as it feels comfortable and calming.

8. **Maintain a steady Pace:** Ensure the movements remain steady and controlled throughout the workout, and prevent abrupt or jerky gestures.

9. **Focus on Relaxation:** Pay attention to how your shoulders feel as you execute the exercise. The objective is to reduce tension and promote relaxation in the shoulder and neck region.

10. **Finish with excellent Posture:** After completing the shoulder shrugs, stand or sit with excellent posture, relax your shoulders down, and take a minute to breathe deeply and feel the relaxation in your upper body.

Shoulder shrugs are a fast and efficient approach to alleviate shoulder and upper back tension. They may be done throughout the day as required to reduce pain. However, if you encounter pain or discomfort during the workout, stop immediately and talk with your healthcare physician. Additionally, if you have any underlying medical illnesses or concerns, obtaining assistance from your healthcare professional before beginning or maintaining any fitness regimen during pregnancy is a good idea.

Arm Circles

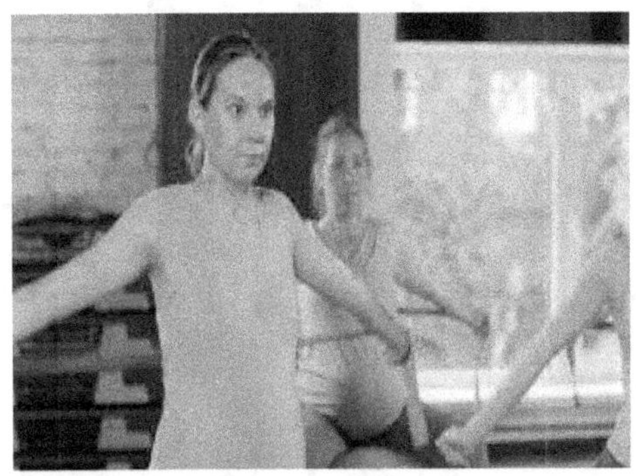

Arm circles are a moderate and effective exercise that may assist pregnant women in improving shoulder mobility, decreasing stress in the upper body, and promoting circulation. Here's how to execute arm circles safely during pregnancy:

Instructions:

1. **Stand or Sit Comfortably:** Find a comfortable and stable sitting or standing posture. Ensure that your feet are hip-width apart if you're standing and your back is well-supported if you're seated.

2. **Relax Your Arms:** Let your arms hang naturally at your sides, with your palms facing down. Keep your hands relaxed.

3. **Engage Your Core:** Gently engage your abdominal muscles to support your lower back and maintain excellent posture.

4. **Begin the Arm Circles:** Inhale deeply, and as you exhale, start creating tiny, controlled circles with your

arms. Imagine creating little circles with your fingers in the
air.

5. **Gradually Increase the Circle Size:** After a few seconds
   of forming little circles, gradually increase the size of the
   circles. Continue to breathe gently and rhythmically.

6. **Continue for 15-30 Seconds:** Keep the arm circles
   continuing for around 15 to 30 seconds, or as long as it
   feels comfortable. Focus on the fluency of the movement
   and the relaxation in your shoulders.

7. **Reverse the Direction:** After the specified time, reverse
   the direction of the arm circles. If you were initially
   drawing circles ahead, switch to producing circles
   backward, and vice versa.

8. **Continue for Another 15-30 Seconds:** Oppositely
   repeat the arm circles for around 15 to 30 seconds.
   Ensure that the motions are slow and controlled.

9. **Maintain a calm tempo:** Maintain a calm and controlled
   tempo throughout the workout, avoiding abrupt or jerky
   actions.

10. **Finish with excellent Posture:** After completing the arm
    circles, stand or sit with excellent posture, relax your arms
    down, and take a minute to breathe deeply and feel the
    relaxation in your upper body.

Arm circles are a moderate workout that may help reduce tension and promote relaxation in the shoulder and upper back region. They are perfect for pregnant ladies searching for an easy, pleasant solution to promote shoulder mobility and decrease pain. However, if you encounter pain or discomfort during the workout, stop immediately and talk with your healthcare physician. Additionally, if you have any underlying medical illnesses or concerns, obtaining assistance from your healthcare professional before beginning or maintaining any fitness regimen during pregnancy is essential.

Hip Circles

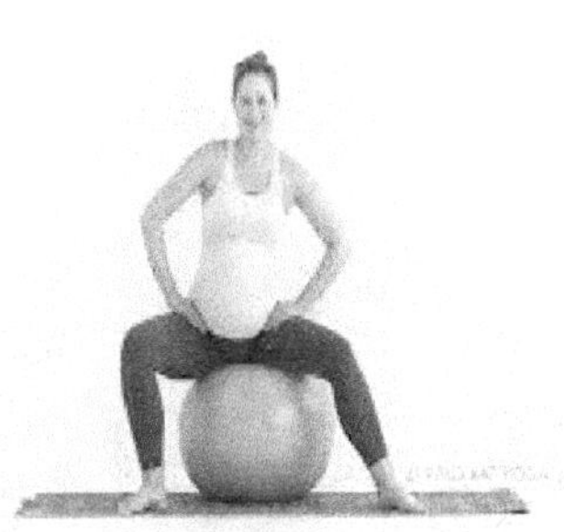

Hip circles are a mild and effective exercise that may assist pregnant women in increasing hip mobility, alleviating stress in the lower back and hips, and enhancing comfort during pregnancy. Here's how to execute hip circles safely during pregnancy:

Instructions:

1. **Stand Comfortably:** Find a comfortable and stable stance with your feet approximately hip-width apart. Ensure your posture is erect and your knees are slightly bent.

2. **Engage Your Core:** Gently engage your abdominal muscles to support your lower back and maintain excellent posture.

3. **Relax Your Arms:** Allow your arms to hang naturally at your sides, keeping your hands relaxed.

4. **Start the Hip Circles:** Inhale intensely, and as you exhale, begin making slow and controlled circular movements with your hips. Imagine drawing a circle with your hips in front of you.

5. **Circle to the Right:** To start, softly push your hips forward, then shift them to the right, tuck your tailbone in, move them back, and lastly, bring them to the left to complete the circle. Continue the circular motion in this direction.

6. **Continue for 15-30 Seconds:** Keep the hip circles running for around 15 to 30 seconds, or as long as it feels comfortable. Focus on the flow of the movement and the relaxation in your lower back and hips.

7. **Reverse the Direction:** After the specified time, reverse the direction of the hip circles. If you initially circled to the right, switch to circling to the left, and vice versa.

8. **Continue for Another 15-30 Seconds:** Oppositely repeat the hip circles for around 15 to 30 seconds. Ensure that the motions are slow and controlled.

9. **Maintain a calm tempo:** Maintain a calm and controlled tempo throughout the workout, avoiding abrupt or jerky actions.

10. **Finish with excellent Posture:** After completing the hip circles, stand with excellent posture, relax your hips, and take a minute to breathe deeply and feel the relaxation in your lower back and hips.

Hip circles may be a calming and helpful exercise for pregnant women, particularly those feeling pain or tension in the hip and lower back regions. However, if you encounter pain or discomfort during the workout, stop immediately and talk with your healthcare physician. Additionally, if you have any underlying medical illnesses or concerns, obtaining assistance from your healthcare professional before beginning or maintaining any fitness regimen during pregnancy is essential.

Leg Swings

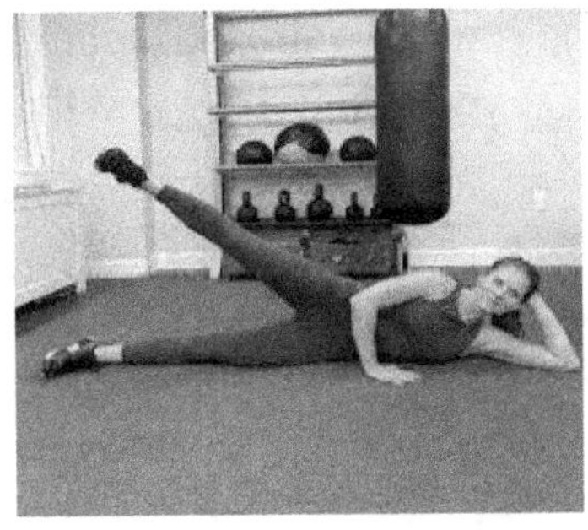

Mobility in your hip and leg muscles. This exercise is excellent for pregnant women and may be especially good for alleviating stress and boosting comfort in the lower body. Here's how to execute leg swings safely during pregnancy:

Instructions:

1. **Find a Supportive Surface:** Stand next to a sturdy surface for support, such as a wall, chair, or countertop. Place one hand loosely on the support for balance.

2. **Stand with Good Posture:** Stand tall with your feet hip-width apart. Ensure that your back is straight and your abdominal muscles are softly engaged to support your lower back.

3. **Hold the Support:** With one hand on the support for balance, softly hold it to maintain stability throughout the exercise.

4. **Swing Your Leg Forward and Backward:** Start with one leg (the right leg) as your beginning leg. Swing your right leg forward in a controlled way, maintaining it straight but not locked at the knee.

5. **Swing Backward:** After swinging your leg forward, gently swing it backward, keeping the same controlled action. You should feel a slight stretch in your hip flexors and the back of your leg.

6. **Repeat for 10-15 Swings:** Continue to swing your leg forth and backward for around 10-15 swings, or as long as it feels comfortable and calming. Keep your motions smooth and rhythmic.

7. **Switch to the Other Leg:** After completing the swings with one leg, switch to the other leg. Perform the same amount of swings with your left leg.

8. **Maintain a calm tempo:** Ensure the leg swings are done at a calm and controlled tempo to prevent abrupt or jerky actions.

9. **Finish with excellent Posture:** After doing leg swings with both legs, stand with excellent posture, relax your legs, and take a minute to breathe deeply and appreciate the enhanced flexibility and relaxation in your hip and leg muscles.

Leg swings are a dynamic stretching exercise that may help alleviate tension in the hip region, enhance relaxation, and improve hip flexibility, which can be particularly advantageous during pregnancy. However, if you encounter pain or discomfort during the workout, stop immediately and talk with your healthcare physician. Additionally, if you have any underlying medical illnesses or concerns, obtaining assistance from your healthcare professional before beginning or maintaining any fitness regimen during pregnancy is essential.

Ankle Circles

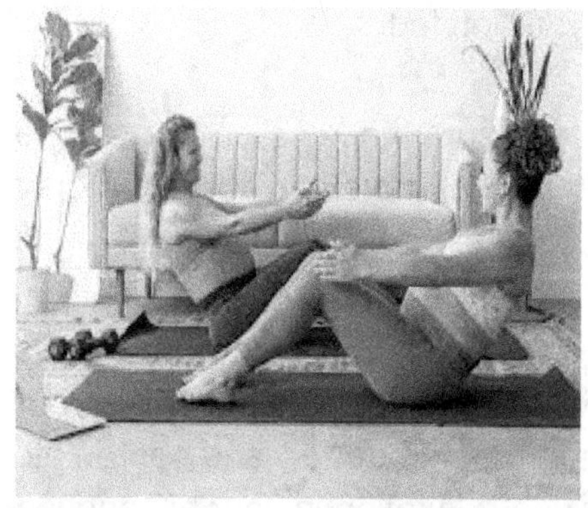

Ankle circles are a simple and effective exercise to enhance ankle mobility, decrease stiffness, and stimulate circulation in the lower legs. These exercises are typically safe during pregnancy and may help ease pain in the ankles and lower legs, which can be prevalent owing to changes in posture and weight distribution. Here's how to practice ankle circles safely during pregnancy:

Instructions:

1. **Sit Comfortably:** Find a comfortable and stable sitting posture on a chair or the floor. You can also practice ankle circles while lying on your side if that's more comfortable for you.

2. **Extend One Leg:** If seated, extend one leg straight in front of you, or if laying on your side, keep the leg you're not working on bent at a comfortable angle.

3. **Relax Your Foot:** Keep your foot relaxed and your toes facing upward. Avoid any strain or clutching with your toes.

4. **Begin the Ankle Circle:** With your toes pointing up, gently start making circular movements with your ankle. Imagine drawing a circle with your big toe. You may start by shifting your foot clockwise.

5. **Perform Clockwise Circles:** Make tiny, controlled clockwise circles with your ankle for 10-15 seconds.

6. **Reverse the Direction:** After completing the clockwise rings, reverse the direction. Start creating counterclockwise circles with your ankle.

7. **Perform Counterclockwise Circles:** Continue with the counterclockwise circles for 10-15 seconds.

8. **Switch to the Other Ankle:** After executing ankle circles with one ankle, switch to the other ankle and execute the same exercises. Extend or bend the opposing leg correspondingly.

9. **Maintain a calm speed:** Ensure the ankle circles are completed at a calm and controlled speed, avoiding abrupt or jerky actions.

10. **Finish with Good Posture:** After performing ankle circles with both ankles, sit up or change your stance as required. Take a minute to breathe deeply and appreciate your ankle joints' enhanced mobility and relaxation.

Ankle circles are a moderate exercise that may help decrease stress and soreness in the ankles and lower legs. They are perfect for pregnant ladies seeking an easy, calming solution to enhance ankle mobility and decrease pain. However, if you encounter pain or discomfort during the workout, stop immediately and talk with your healthcare physician. Additionally, if you have any underlying medical illnesses or concerns, obtaining assistance from your healthcare professional before beginning or maintaining any fitness regimen during pregnancy is essential.

Gentle Squats

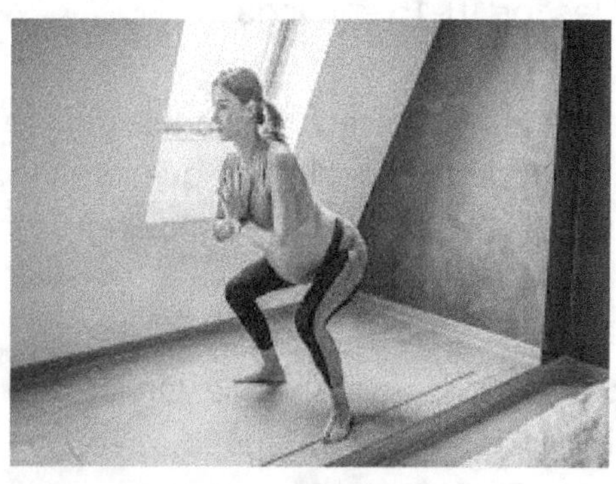

Gentle squats are a safe and effective workout for pregnant women that may help increase lower body strength, balance, and general comfort during pregnancy. Squats can also help prepare your body for the physical demands of labor and delivery. Here's how to conduct gentle squats during pregnancy:

Instructions:

1. **Find a Stable Position:** Stand with your feet shoulder-width apart or slightly wider for stability. You may also use a chair or a wall for support if required.

2. **Engage Your Core:** Gently engage your abdominal muscles to support your lower back and maintain proper posture throughout the activity.

3. **Relax Your Shoulders:** Keep your shoulders relaxed and away from your ears.

4. **Start the Squat:** Inhale deeply, and as you exhale, gently lower your body by bending your knees. Imagine sitting back in an imagined chair.

5. **Lower Gradually:** Lower yourself only as far as you feel comfortable and control the action. It's crucial to avoid squatting too profoundly to prevent overstretching or placing undue strain on the pelvic region.

6. **Knees Over Toes:** Ensure that your knees remain aligned with your toes and do not slide beyond your toes while you squat.

7. **Keep Your Back Straight:** Maintain a straight back throughout the squat. Avoid rounding or arching your lower back.

8. **Stop at the Bottom:** Once you've achieved a comfortable squatting depth, stop for a minute and exhale as you gently return to the beginning position.

9. **Repeat for 10-15 Repetitions:** Perform 10-15 repetitions of mild squats or as many as you feel comfortable with.

Focus on the quality of the movement rather than the quantity.

10. **Utilize Support If Necessary:** If you have difficulty keeping balance or need extra support, you may use a chair or wall for stability. Hold onto the support with your hands while completing the squats.

11. **Finish with Good Posture:** After finishing the squats, stand up straight, relax your legs, and take a minute to breathe deeply.

Gentle squats are:
- It is a fantastic approach to developing leg muscles.
- Preserving lower body mobility.
- Supporting your posture during pregnancy.

They may also help reduce lower back and hip aches. However, if you encounter any pain, dizziness, or discomfort while practicing squats, stop immediately and talk with your healthcare physician. Additionally, if you have any underlying medical illnesses or concerns, obtaining assistance from your healthcare professional before beginning or maintaining any fitness regimen during pregnancy is essential.

Pendulum Arms

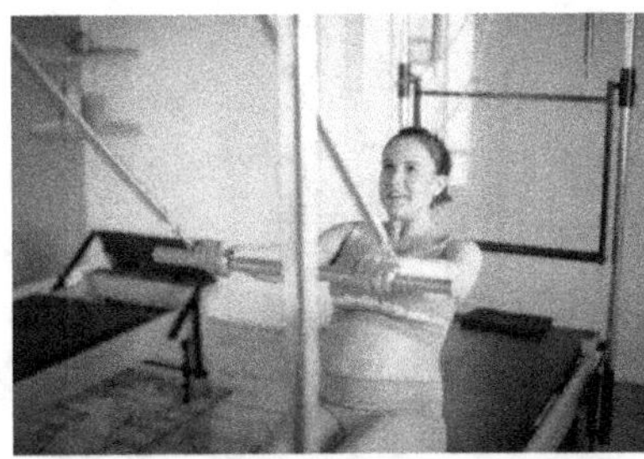

Pendulum arm swings, also known as pendulum arms or arm circles, are a simple and effective exercise to enhance shoulder mobility, ease tension in the upper body, and promote relaxation. This exercise is typically safe for pregnant women and may help ease pain in the shoulder and neck region, which can be frequent during pregnancy owing to changes in posture and weight distribution. Here's how to execute pendulum arms safely during pregnancy:

Instructions:

1. **Stand Comfortably:** Find a comfortable and stable stance with your feet approximately hip-width apart. Ensure your posture is erect and your knees are slightly bent.

2. **Relax Your Arms:** Allow your arms to hang freely at your sides, with your palms facing down. Keep your hands relaxed.

3. **Engage Your Core:** Gently engage your abdominal muscles to support your lower back and maintain excellent posture.

4. **Start the Pendulum Arms:** Inhale deeply, and as you exhale, start making tiny, controlled circular movements

with your arms. Imagine creating little circles with your
fingers in the air.

5. **Gradually Increase the Circle Size:** After a few seconds
   of forming little circles, gradually increase the size of the
   circles. Continue to breathe gently and rhythmically.

6. **Continue for 15-30 Seconds:** Keep the arm circles
   running for around 15 to 30 seconds, or as long as it feels
   comfortable and calming. Focus on the fluency of the
   movement and the relaxation in your shoulders.

7. **Reverse the Direction:** After the specified time, reverse
   the direction of the arm circles. If you were initially
   drawing circles ahead, switch to producing circles
   backward, and vice versa.

8. **Continue for Another 15-30 Seconds:** Oppositely
   repeat the arm circles for around 15 to 30 seconds.
   Ensure that the motions are slow and controlled.

9. **Maintain a calm tempo:** Maintain a calm and controlled
   tempo throughout the workout, avoiding abrupt or jerky
   actions.

10. **Finish with excellent Posture:** After finishing the
    pendulum arms, stand with excellent posture, relax your
    arms down, take a minute to breathe deeply, and
    appreciate the enhanced mobility and relaxation in your
    shoulder and upper body.

Pendulum arms are a moderate workout that may help decrease stress and pain in the shoulder and upper back region. They are perfect for pregnant ladies searching for an easy, pleasant solution to promote shoulder mobility and decrease pain. However, if you encounter pain or discomfort during the workout, stop immediately and talk with your healthcare physician. Additionally, if you have any underlying medical illnesses or concerns, obtaining assistance from your healthcare professional before beginning or maintaining any fitness regimen during pregnancy is essential.

Pregnancy-Safe Core Activation

Pregnancy-safe core activation exercises are vital for maintaining core strength and stability throughout pregnancy while guaranteeing the mother's and baby's safety. Traditional core workouts like crunches and planks may be changed to make them suitable for pregnancy. Here's how to practice pregnancy-safe core activation exercises:

Pelvic Tilts

Pelvic tilts stimulate and develop the deep abdominal muscles without placing undue strain on the abdomen.

Instructions:
1. **Stand or Sit:** Find a comfortable and steady sitting or standing posture.

2. **Engage Your Core:** Encourage your deep abdominal muscles by bringing your navel toward your spine. Imagine moving your pelvis slightly forward.

3. **Hold and Release:** Hold this posture for a few seconds while breathing normally, then release. Repeat the exercise for 10-15 times.

Seated Marching

Seated marching is a healthy approach to working your core muscles while seated.

Instructions:
- **Sit Comfortably:** Sit on a chair with your feet flat on the floor, hip-width apart.

- **Engage Your Core:** Encourage your deep abdominal muscles by bringing your navel toward your spine.

March in Place

Instructions:
1. While maintaining core engagement, elevate one knee as though you're marching in place.
2. Lower it, and then elevate the opposite knee.
3. Continue this action for 10-15 times on each leg.

Standing Marching

Standing marching is another approach to working your core while standing.

Instructions:
1. **Stand Tall:** Find a comfortable and sturdy stance with your feet hip-width apart.

2. **Engage Your Core:** Encourage your deep abdominal muscles by bringing your navel toward your spine.

March in Place:
1. Lift one knee as though you're marching in place.
2. Lower it, and then elevate the opposite knee.
3. Continue this action for 10-15 times on each leg.

Diaphragmatic Breathing with Core Engagement:
Diaphragmatic breathing mixed with core engagement helps strengthen the deep abdominal muscles and promotes relaxation.

Instructions:
1. **Sit or Lie Down:** Find a comfortable sitting or lying posture.

2. **Engage Your Core:** Encourage your deep abdominal muscles by bringing your navel toward your spine.

3. **Deep Breathing:** Inhale deeply through your nose, allowing your belly to rise as you fill your lungs with air. Exhale gently through your lips, continuing to activate your core muscles.

4. **Repeat:** Practice deep diaphragmatic breathing with core engagement for a few minutes, concentrating on the relaxation and activation of your core muscles.

These pregnancy-safe core activation exercises help you maintain core strength and stability while decreasing the danger of diastasis recti (separation of the abdominal muscles). However, talking with your healthcare practitioner before beginning or maintaining any fitness regimen during pregnancy is vital, particularly if you have any underlying medical issues or concerns. Your healthcare professional may give specific counsel based on your unique requirements and pregnancy stage.

Cool-Down Exercises

Deep Breathing

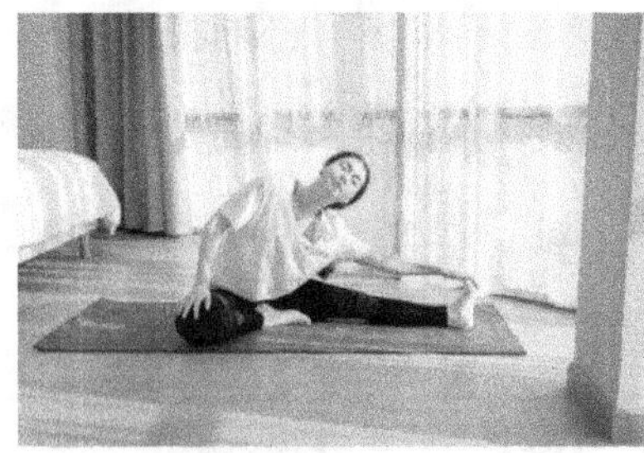

Deep breathing, also known as diaphragmatic or abdominal breathing, is a relaxation and stress-reduction method that utilizes your diaphragm to take slow, deep breaths. It may be beneficial during pregnancy to decrease stress, enhance oxygen flow to both you and your baby, and induce relaxation. Here's how to practice deep breathing:

Instructions:

1. **Find a Comfortable Position:** Sit or lie in a comfortable and peaceful spot where you won't be disturbed.

2. **Relax Your Body:** Close your eyes and take a minute to relax your muscles, beginning from your toes and working your way up to your head. Release whatever stress you may be harboring.

3. **Place Your Hands:** Place one hand on your chest and the other on your belly, right below your ribs.

4. **Inhale Slowly:** Inhale through your nose slowly and deeply, allowing your belly to rise as you fill your lungs with air. Your chest should stay reasonably motionless throughout this time.

5. **Exhale Slowly:** Exhale through your mouth slowly and thoroughly, allowing your belly to sink as you remove air from your lungs.

6. **Focus on Your Breath:** Concentrate on your breath as you inhale and exhale softly. Pay attention to the rise and fall of your belly rather than the movement of your chest.

7. **Count Your Breath:** You may count the duration of your inhales and exhales to assist in regulating your breath. For example, inhale for a count of four, hold momentarily, and then exhale for a count of four. Adjust the count to what feels comfortable for you.

8. **Maintain a Rhythmic Pattern:** Establish a rhythmic pattern of breathing that is comfortable and relaxing for you. Focus on making your exhales slightly longer than your inhales since this might increase relaxation.

9. **Empty Your thoughts:** As you breathe deeply, attempt to empty your thoughts of any distractions or problems. Focus exclusively on your breath and the sense of tranquility.

10. **Practice for Several Minutes:** Continue to practice deep breathing for several minutes, preferably 5-10 minutes or more if you have the time.

11. **Gradual Return:** When ready to end, take a few normal breaths and gradually return to your usual breathing rhythm. Open your eyes and sit up carefully as if you were lying down.

Deep breathing may be performed during pregnancy to decrease stress, control anxiety, and promote relaxation. It may also be highly beneficial during labor and delivery to reduce pain and anxiety. Regular practice of deep breathing may give several advantages for both you and your kid.

Static Stretches

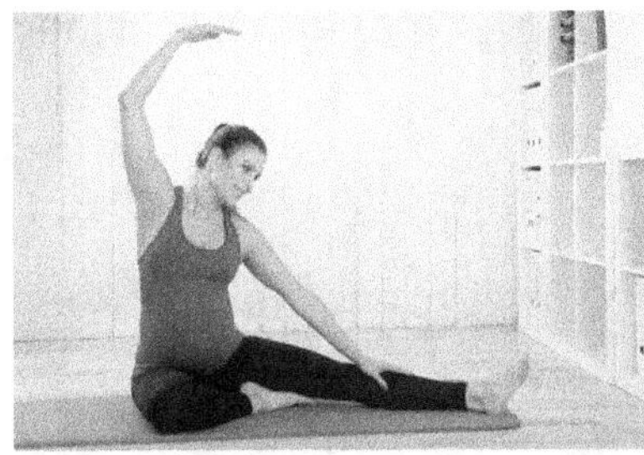 Static stretches are an effective technique for pregnant women to develop flexibility, decrease muscular tension, and relieve pain. These stretches should be done slowly and gently, and they may be especially effective for resolving common pregnancy-related concerns, including lower back discomfort, hip stiffness, and leg cramps. Here are several safe and effective static stretches for pregnant women:

1. Seated Forward Bend:

This stretch helps ease discomfort and extends the hamstrings and lower back.

Instructions:

- Sit on the floor with your legs outstretched.
- Gently bend at your hips and stretch forward toward your toes.
- Keep your back straight and go as far as is comfortable.
- Hold the stretch for 15-30 seconds and then gently release.

2. Hip Flexor Stretch:

This stretch targets the hip flexors, which may get stiff during pregnancy.

Instructions:
- Kneel on the floor with one foot in front and the other knee behind you.
- Shift your weight slightly forward to experience a modest stretch in the hip of the rear leg.
- Hold for 15-30 seconds and switch to the other side.

3. Cat-Cow Stretch:

This yoga-inspired stretch helps with spinal flexibility and reduces stress in the lower back.

Instructions:
- Get on your hands and knees in a tabletop posture.
- Inhale as you arch your back (Cow posture), raising your head and tailbone.
- Exhale as you curve your back (Cat position), tucking your chin and tailbone.
- Repeat this exercise for 15-30 seconds, flowing with your breath.

4. Butterfly Stretch:

This stretch targets the inner thighs and groin muscles.

Instructions:

- Sit on the floor with your feet together and knees bent outward.
- Gently push your knees toward the floor using your elbows.
- Hold for 15-30 seconds, experiencing a slight stretch in the inner thighs.

5. Child's Pose:

This soothing stretch helps ease lower back discomfort and promotes relaxation.

Instructions:

- Kneel on the floor and sit back on your heels.
- Extend your arms forward and drop your chest toward the floor.
- Rest your forehead on the ground or a pillow.
- Hold for 15-30 seconds while inhaling deeply.

6. Quadriceps Stretch:

This stretch targets the front thigh muscles (quadriceps).

Instructions:

- Stand with one hand on a support (e.g., a wall or chair) for balance.
- Bend one knee and grip your ankle behind you with your hand.

- Gently draw your heel toward your buttocks while keeping your knees close together.
- Hold for 15-30 seconds, and then swap legs.

7. Calf Stretch:

This stretch targets the calf muscles, which may get stiff during pregnancy.

Instructions:
- Stand facing a wall, with one foot forward and one foot back.
- Place your hands on the wall and bend forward, keeping your back heel on the ground.
- Feel a slight stretch in the calf of the rear leg.
- Hold for 15-30 seconds and swap legs.

Perform these static stretches periodically to help increase your flexibility, decrease muscular tension, and promote calm during pregnancy. Always listen to your body; if you suffer pain or discomfort when stretching, stop immediately and talk with your healthcare professional. Also, contact your healthcare professional before beginning or maintaining any exercise or stretching regimen during pregnancy, particularly if you have any underlying medical disorders or concerns.

Cat-Cow Stretch

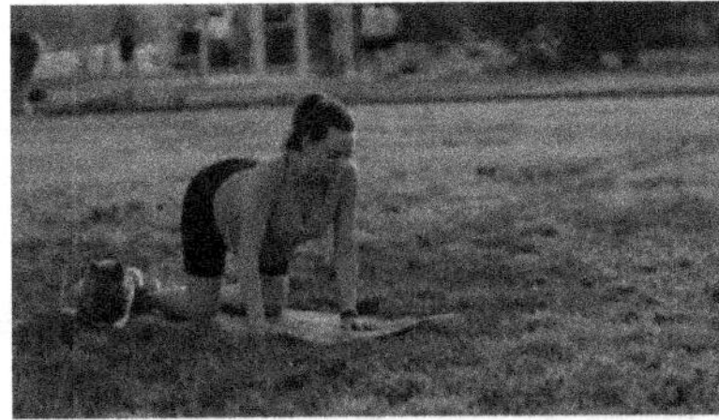

The Cat-Cow stretch is a moderate and effective yoga-inspired stretch that may be useful for pregnant women. It helps increase spinal flexibility, reduce stress in the lower back, and promote relaxation. This stretch is especially effective during pregnancy to relieve frequent discomforts linked with changes in posture and weight distribution. Here's how to execute the Cat-Cow stretch safely during pregnancy:

Instructions:

1. Get on Your Hands and Knees
- Start in a tabletop posture on the floor.
- Place your hands strictly under your shoulders and your knees under your hips.
- Ensure your wrists are aligned with your shoulders and your legs are hip-width apart.

2. **Engage Your Core:** Encourage your abdominal muscles to support your lower back.

3. **Begin with Cow Pose (Inhale):** Inhale deeply, arch your back and raise your head and tailbone upward. Allow your tummy to descend toward the floor, producing a concave curve in your lower Back. Lift your head, facing slightly upward or forward.

4. **Transition to Cat Pose (Exhale):** Exhale gently as you curve your back like a cat, bringing your chin into your chest and tucking your pelvis beneath. Feel the strain along your spine as it curls upward.

5. **Repeat the Movement:** Continue to move between Cow Pose and Cat Pose with your breath. Inhale as you arch your back, elevate your head for Cow Pose, and exhale as you circle your back and tuck your chin for Cat Pose.

6. **Perform for 30 Seconds to 1 Minute:** Repeat the Cat-Cow stretch for around 30 seconds to 1 minute or as long as it feels comfortable and peaceful.

7. **Maintain a gradual Pace:** Ensure that the motions are gradual and controlled, and concentrate on the smoothness of the stretch and the relaxation in your lower back.

8. **Finish with a Neutral Spine:** After finishing the stretch, return to a neutral tabletop posture with your back flat.

The Cat-Cow stretch is a gentle approach to ease stress in the lower back, enhance spinal flexibility, and induce relaxation during pregnancy. It may also aid with improving posture and alleviating pain linked with pregnancy-related changes. However, if you encounter pain or discomfort during the workout, stop immediately and talk with your healthcare physician. Additionally, if you have any underlying medical illnesses or concerns, obtaining assistance from your healthcare professional before beginning or maintaining any workout or stretching regimen during pregnancy is essential.

Child's Pose

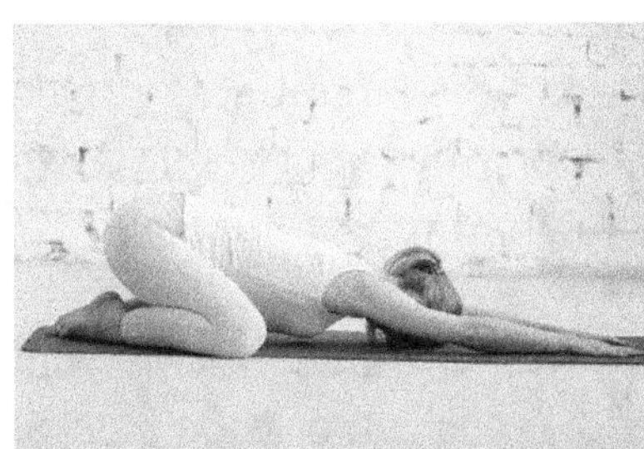

Child's Pose is a peaceful and mild yoga stretch that may be customized for pregnant women to encourage relaxation, reduce lower back stiffness, and lessen discomfort. It's a pleasant resting posture that helps you to take a break and discover a feeling of serenity throughout pregnancy. Here's how to execute a Child's Pose safely during pregnancy:

Instructions:

1. **Start in a Kneeling posture:** Begin on your hands and knees in a tabletop posture. Ensure that your wrists are aligned with your shoulders and your legs are hip-width apart.

2. **Create a Wide Knee Position:** Separate your knees slightly wider than hip-width apart to allow space for your increasing tummy. This alteration avoids any pressure on your abdomen.

3. **Engage Your Core:** Gently engage your abdominal muscles to support your lower back and maintain excellent posture.

4. **Sit Back on Your Heels:** Slowly rotate your hips backward, pushing your buttocks toward your heels. This movement should feel mild and comforting. If your hips don't comfortably reach your heels, that's OK; go only as far as feels comfortable.

5. **Stretch Your Arms Forward:** As you sit back, stretch your arms forward along the floor. Keep your hands down and your fingers stretching out from you.

6. **Rest Your Forehead on the Ground:** Allow your forehead to rest on the floor or a cushion or yoga block if required. This gives further comfort and support for your head and neck.

7. **Breathe Deeply:** Take slow, deep breaths in this posture. Feel your belly expand as you inhale, and let go of any tension in your body as you exhale.

8. **Hold for 1-2 Minutes:** Remain in Child's Pose for 1-2 minutes or as long as it feels comfortable. Focus on relaxation and deep breathing.

9. **To Come Out of the posture:** To leave the posture, slowly move your hands back toward your body and use your hands for support while you pull your upper body away from your legs. Return to a sitting posture and then rise gently if desired.

Child's Pose during pregnancy may be a calming and peaceful stretch that delivers a feeling of relaxation and release from the physical rigors of pregnancy. It helps you connect with your breath and rest when required if you encounter discomfort or suffering while in the Child's Pose, change your posture, or come out of it. As with any workout or stretch during pregnancy, you must contact your healthcare professional before beginning or maintaining any regimen, particularly if you have any underlying medical issues or concerns.

Hip Flexor Stretch

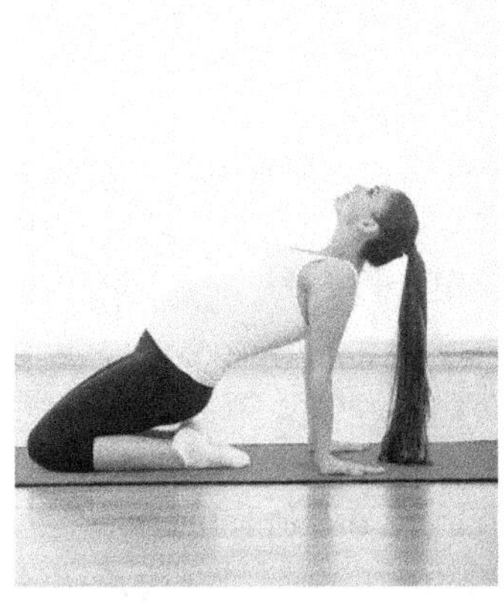

Stretching the hip flexors may be advantageous for pregnant women since these muscles can become tight owing to changes in posture and weight distribution. Here's how to execute a hip flexor stretch safely during pregnancy:

Kneeling Hip Flexor Stretch:

This stretch may reduce tension in the hip flexor muscles and increase comfort.

Instructions:

1. **Find a Comfortable Surface:** Begin by kneeling on a comfortable and supporting surface, such as a yoga mat or cushion. Place a soft surface beneath your knees for increased comfort if required.

2. **Knee and Hip Alignment:** posture your knees under your hips and your hands under your shoulders in a tabletop posture. Ensure that your wrists are aligned with your shoulders and your legs are hip-width apart.

3. **Engage Your Core:** Gently engage your abdominal muscles to support your lower back and maintain excellent posture.

4. **Step One Foot Forward:** Take one foot and step it forward, setting it flat on the floor in front of you. Your knee should be at a 90-degree angle.

5. **Transfer Your Weight Forward:** Gently transfer your weight forward, leaning into the hip flexor stretch. You should feel a slight stretch at the front of the hip and thigh of the outstretched leg.

6. **Tuck Your Tailbone:** Tuck your tailbone gently under and engage your glutes to deepen the stretch. This motion promotes the stretch in the hip flexor.

7. **Hold the Stretch:** Hold the stretch for 15-30 seconds or longer if it feels comfortable and peaceful. Focus on relaxation and deep breathing.

8. **Move to the Other Leg:** After holding the stretch on one side, gently return to the beginning position and move to the other leg. Step the opposing foot forward and repeat the stretch on the other side.

9. **Maintain a calm speed:** Ensure the stretch is completed at a calm and controlled speed, avoiding abrupt or jerky movements.

10. **Finish with Good Posture:** Return to a tabletop posture with your back flat after completing the stretch on both sides.

The kneeling hip flexor stretch is a healthy approach to relieving tight hip flexor muscles during pregnancy. It helps ease stress and soreness in the front of the hip and thigh region. However, if you encounter pain or discomfort during the workout, stop immediately and talk with your healthcare physician. As with any workout or stretch during pregnancy, obtaining assistance from your healthcare professional before beginning or maintaining any regimen is essential, particularly if you have any underlying medical issues or concerns is essential.

Inner Thigh Stretch

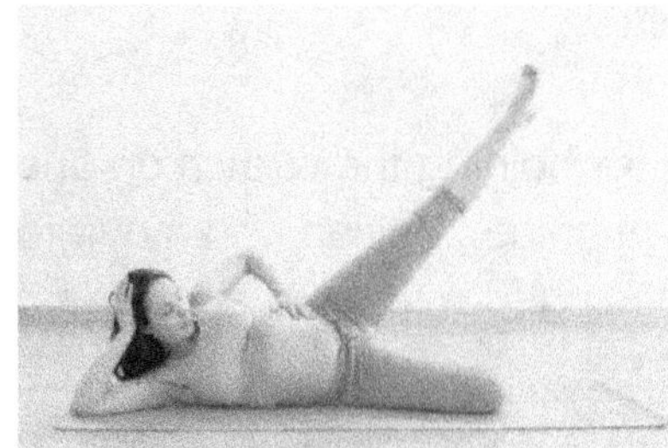

Stretching the inner thighs may help ease stress and pain during pregnancy, particularly when the body experiences weight distribution and posture changes. Here's how to execute an inner thigh stretch safely during pregnancy:

Seated Inner Thigh Stretch:

This stretch may assist in targeting the inner thigh muscles (adductors) and encourage relaxation.

Instructions:

1. **Find a Comfortable Seat:** Sit on the floor with your back straight and your legs in front of you.

2. **Bend Your Knees:** Bend your knees and bring the soles of your feet together, allowing your knees to extend outward. This will produce a diamond shape with your legs.

3. **Hold Your Feet:** Hold your feet with your hands. Depending on your flexibility and comfort, you can clasp your ankles or hold your toes.

4. **Engage Your Core:** Gently engage your abdominal muscles to support your lower back and maintain excellent posture.

5. **Relax Your Hips:** Allow your knees to descend toward the floor, experiencing a stretch along the inner thighs. It's vital to go just as far as is comfortable for you, and there's no need to push your knees down.

6. **Hold the Stretch:** Hold the stretch for 15-30 seconds or longer if it feels comfortable and peaceful. Focus on relaxation and deep breathing.

7. **Maintain a Straight Back:** Throughout the stretch, ensure that your back stays straight and your chest is open. Avoid rounding your back.

8. **Gently Release:** To come out of the stretch, release your feet and gently pull your knees together.

9. **Finish with Good Posture:** Return to a sitting posture with your legs extended, and take a minute to breathe deeply.

The sitting inner thigh stretch is a gentle method to target the inner thigh muscles and induce relaxation. It's vital to complete the stretch with control and avoid violent movements. Stop immediately and talk with your healthcare professional if you encounter any pain or discomfort throughout the activity. As with any workout or stretch during pregnancy, obtaining assistance from your healthcare professional before beginning or maintaining any regimen is essential, particularly if you have any underlying medical issues or concerns is essential.

Chest Opener

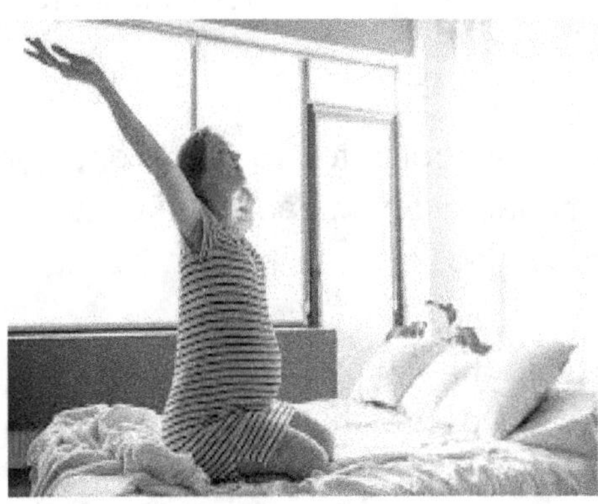

The chest opening stretch is a good exercise for pregnant women, as it helps prevent the curving of the shoulders and upper back that might develop owing to changes in posture during pregnancy. It also promotes improved breathing and relaxation. Here's how to conduct a chest opening stretch:

Instructions:

1. **Find a Comfortable Standing Position:** Stand tall with your feet hip-width apart. Ensure you are on a sturdy surface.

2. **Engage Your Core:** Gently engage your abdominal muscles to support your lower back and maintain excellent posture.

3. **Interlace Your Fingers:** Reach your arms behind your back and interlace your fingers. If this is unpleasant, you may use a towel or yoga strap to grasp onto instead.

4. **Open Your Chest:** While maintaining your arms straight, gently pull your interlaced hands or the strap upward and slightly backward, opening your chest. This action should feel like you're dragging your shoulder blades toward each other.

5. **Lift Your Chest:** As you open your chest, lift your chin slightly. This helps maintain a straight neck position.

6. **Hold the Stretch:** Hold the stretch for 15-30 seconds or longer if it feels comfortable and peaceful. Focus on relaxation and deep breathing.

7. **Maintain Good Posture:** Ensure that your back stays straight and your shoulders are relaxed throughout the stretch. Avoid arching your lower back.

8. **Remove Your Hands:** Gently remove your interlaced fingers or the strap, bringing your arms back to your sides.

9. **Finish with Good Posture:** Stand with your back straight shoulders relaxed, and take a minute to breathe deeply.

The chest opener stretch is a moderate approach to offset bad posture and improve chest and shoulder openness. It may be beneficial during pregnancy when the increasing belly might contribute to rounded shoulders. Stop immediately and talk with your healthcare professional if you encounter any pain or discomfort throughout the activity. As with any workout or stretch during pregnancy, obtaining assistance from your healthcare professional before beginning or maintaining any regimen is essential, particularly if you have any underlying medical issues or concerns is essential.

Heel to Buttock Stretch

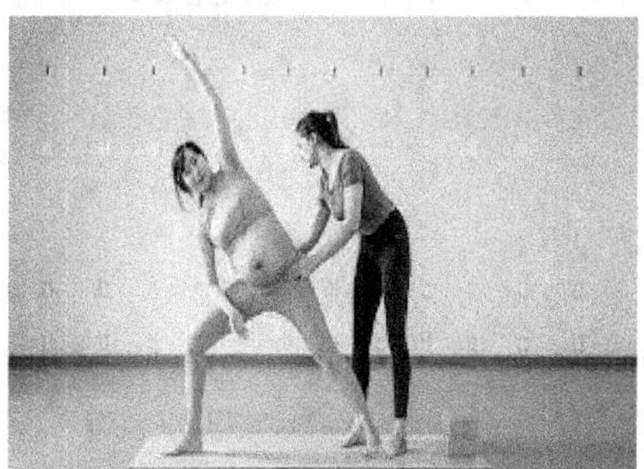

The heel-to-buttock stretch, also known as a quadriceps stretch, may be suitable for pregnant women to release tension in the front thigh muscles (quadriceps) and enhance flexibility. This stretch may help ease pain in the hip and thigh region, which is typical during pregnancy owing to changes in posture and weight distribution. Here's how to conduct the heel-to-buttock stretch safely during pregnancy:

Instructions:

1. **Find a Comfortable Surface:** Begin by standing in a comfortable and supporting stance. You may utilize a wall or a chair for balance if required.

2. **Engage Your Core:** Gently engage your abdominal muscles to support your lower back and maintain excellent posture.

3. **Shift Your Weight:** Shift your weight to one leg while maintaining your back straight.

4. **Bend Your Knee:** Bend your other knee and put your heel closer to your buttock.

5. **Reach for Your Foot:** Reach behind you with the hand on the same side as the bent leg. Grab your ankle or foot lightly.

6. **Gently Bring Your Heel:** Use your hand to bring your heel closer to your buttock gently. You should feel a stretch at the front of your thigh (quadriceps).

7. **Maintain Good Posture:** Ensure that your back stays straight and your chest is open throughout the stretch. Avoid arching your lower back.

8. **Hold the Stretch:** Hold the stretch for 15-30 seconds or longer if it feels comfortable and peaceful. Focus on relaxation and deep breathing.

9. **Gently Release:** Slowly release your foot and return it to the ground.

Switch to the Other Leg:

- Repeat the stretch on the other leg.
- Shift your weight to the other leg, bend the knee, and bring the heel toward the buttock.
- Reach for your foot and gradually move it closer to your buttock.

10. **Finish with Good Posture:** Stand with your back straight shoulders relaxed, and take a minute to breathe deeply.

The heel-to-buttock stretch may help reduce stress in the quadriceps and increase flexibility during pregnancy. However, if you encounter pain or discomfort during the workout, stop immediately and talk with your healthcare physician. As with any workout or stretch during pregnancy, obtaining assistance from your healthcare professional before beginning or maintaining any regimen is essential, particularly if you have any underlying medical issues or concerns is essential.

Full-Body Relaxation

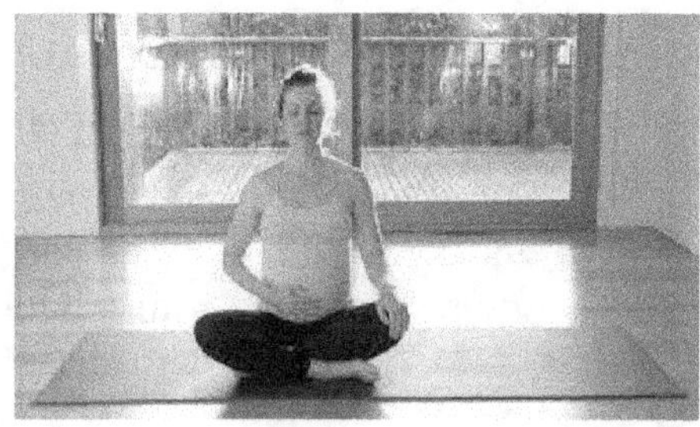

Full-body relaxation is a crucial technique throughout pregnancy to decrease stress, increase physical comfort, and prepare your body for the changes it's experiencing.

Here's a step-by-step tutorial on how to attain full-body relaxation:

Instructions:
1. **Find a Quiet area:** Choose a quiet and comfortable area where you won't be bothered. Depending on what feels best for you, you may lay down on a comfortable surface, such as a yoga mat, bed, or sofa, or sit in a comfy chair.

2. **Get Comfortable:** If lying down, use a cushion to support your head and another pillow under your knees for increased comfort. Ensure your body is well-supported.

3. **Close Your Eyes:** Close your eyes to reduce visual distractions and produce a more profound sensation of relaxation.

4. **Progressive Muscle Relaxation:** Start at your toes and work your way up, slowly relaxing each muscle group. Begin by concentrating on your toes, feet, ankles, and so on, progressing up your body. As you concentrate on each muscle area, intentionally release any stress or stiffness you may harbor.

5. **Deep Breathing:**
- Take slow, deep breaths in through your nose and exhale gently through your mouth.
- Focus on the rhythm of your breath.
- Inhale deeply, allowing your abdomen to rise, and exhale completely, releasing tension with each breath.

6. **Visualize calm:** Imagine a wave of calm flowing through your body with each breath. Visualize warmth and contentment extending from the top of your head to the tips of your toes.

7. **Scan Your Body:** Mentally scan your body to check for any areas of tension or pain. If you detect any, concentrate on those locations and intentionally release the tension with your breath.

8. **Relax Your Jaw:** Release any tightness in your jaw by allowing your teeth to separate slightly. Allow your face muscles to relax, including your forehead, cheeks, and neck.

9. **Mental imaging:** Use mental imaging to take oneself to a pleasant and serene area, whether a beach, a forest, or a peaceful meadow. Imagine that area's sights, sounds, and feelings, and let it fill you with a sense of tranquility.

10. **Let Go of Ideas:** If your mind begins to wander or is flooded with ideas, notice them without judgment and gently return your concentration to your breath and relaxation.

11. **Stay in This State:** Remain calm for as long as you wish, whether a few minutes or longer. Allow yourself to appreciate the profound sensation of serenity and relaxation.

12. Awaken Slowly:

- Do so gently when you're ready to quit the relaxation exercise.
- Start wiggling your fingers and toes, then slowly move your limbs.
- Stretch your body and open your eyes gently.

Full-body relaxation may be done daily or as frequently as you wish to manage stress, alleviate physical pain, and increase general well-being throughout pregnancy. Regular relaxation methods might help to a healthier and more pleas ant pregnancy experience.

CHAPTER FOUR

Cardiovascular Exercises for Expectant Moms

Walking

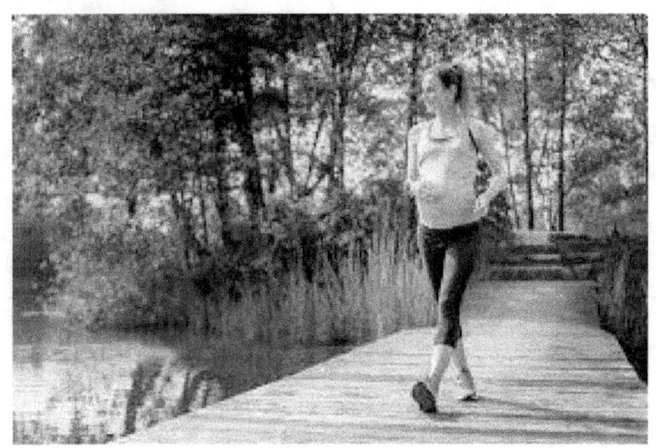

Walking is one of the most accessible and safe kinds of exercise for pregnant women, and it delivers various advantages throughout pregnancy. It helps maintain overall fitness, supports healthy weight growth, enhances mood, and stimulates circulation. Here are some recommendations and guidelines for walking during pregnancy:

1. speak with Your Healthcare practitioner: Before commencing any exercise regimen during pregnancy, including walking, speak with your healthcare practitioner. They may make specific advice depending on your unique health and pregnancy status.

2. Choose Supportive Footwear: Wear comfortable walking shoes with solid arch support. This will help lower the likelihood of foot and leg pain.

3. Dress Comfortably: Wear loose-fitting, breathable clothes that allow for flexibility of movement. Layer garments as required to adjust to changing weather conditions.

4. Be hydrated: Drink lots of water before, during, and after your walk to be well-hydrated. Dehydration might raise the risk of overheating.

5. Warm-Up: Start with a simple warm-up to prepare your muscles and joints for activity. Perform some mild stretching and deep breathing.

6. Maintain Good Posture: Stand up straight with your shoulders back and your head aligned with your spine. Engage your core muscles softly to support your lower back.

7. speed Yourself: Walk at a speed that permits you to carry on a conversation comfortably. You should be able to converse without getting winded.

8. Use Proper Walking Technique: Strike the ground with your heel, roll through the arch of your foot, and push off with your toes. This helps lessen the impact on your joints.

9. Listen to Your Body: Pay attention to how you feel throughout your stroll. Slow down or stop immediately if you encounter any pain, dizziness, shortness of breath, or discomfort.

10. Include mild Stretches: Do mild stretching activities to enhance flexibility and alleviate muscular stress after your stroll.

11. Stay Safe: Choose well-lit, safe walking routes, mainly if you walk in the evening or early morning. If you walk on uneven ground, be particularly careful.

12. Be Mindful of Balance: Your center of gravity may alter as your pregnancy advances. Be cautious of your balance and use additional caution while walking on slick terrain.

13. Monitor Your Heart Rate: Avoid overexertion by maintaining your heart rate within a reasonable range. Aim for a heart rate that permits you to communicate comfortably.

14. Stay Cool: On hot days, walk at cooler periods, such as early morning or late evening, to minimize overheating. Wear a wide-brimmed hat and apply sunscreen.

15. relax When Needed: Don't hesitate to pause and relax if you feel weary or exhausted.

Walking during pregnancy is typically safe and healthy, but it's crucial to be careful and emphasize your comfort and well-being. If you have concerns or suffer odd symptoms while walking, check with your healthcare physician soon. They can give direction and ensure that walking stays a safe and fun part of your pregnancy routine.

Swimming

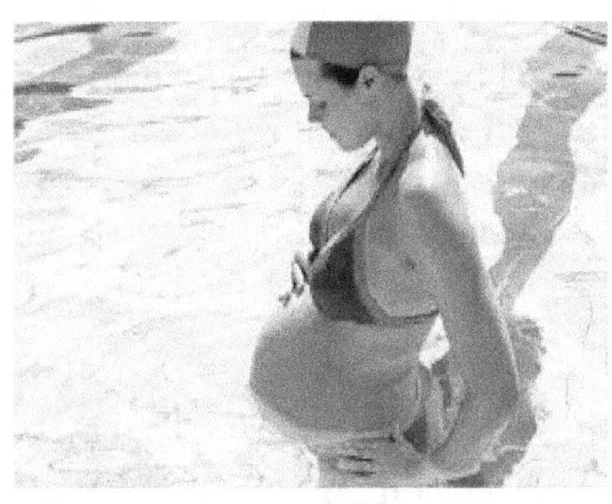

Swimming is a beautiful fitness choice for pregnant women since it delivers a full-body workout while being easy on the joints. It provides many advantages, including better cardiovascular fitness, less edema, alleviation of back pain, and greater relaxation. Here are some advice and rules for swimming during pregnancy:

1. Speak with Your Healthcare practitioner: Before beginning or maintaining a swimming regimen during pregnancy, speak with your healthcare practitioner. They may analyze your particular health and pregnancy status and give advice.

2. Choose a Safe Environment: Swim in a well-maintained and frequently treated pool to guarantee adequate water quality. Avoid swimming in open bodies of water, such as lakes or rivers, owing to possible waterborne dangers.

3. Select a Supportive swimwear: Invest in comfortable and supportive maternity swimwear that supports your developing belly and gives sufficient covering and support.

4. Be hydrated: Drink lots of water before, during, and after your swim to be well-hydrated. Dehydration might raise the risk of overheating.

5. Warm-Up: Start with a simple warm-up by strolling in the water and completing some light stretching exercises to prepare your muscles and joints.

6. **Pay Attention to Pool Temperature:** Choose a pool with a pleasant water temperature, often about 84-86°F (29-30°C). Hot tubs and pools should be avoided since they might contribute to hyperthermia.

7. **Maintain excellent Posture:** While swimming, maintain excellent posture. Engage your core muscles softly to support your lower back and preserve alignment.

8. **Swim at Your rate: S**wim at a comfortable rate that enables you to enjoy the sport without feeling breathless. You should be able to hold a conversation while swimming.

9. **Adopt appropriate Swimming Technique:** If you are an experienced swimmer, adopt appropriate swimming strokes and techniques. Avoid excessive twisting or turning motions.

10. **Listen to Your Body:** Heed your body's messages. If you encounter any pain, dizziness, shortness of breath, or discomfort, pause and relax.

11. **Include flotation equipment:** If required, utilize flotation equipment such as swim noodles or a kickboard to aid with buoyancy and stability in the water.

12. **moderate Stretches:** After swimming, do moderate stretching activities to enhance flexibility and minimize muscular tension.

13. **Safety:** Always swim in a pool with a lifeguard or have someone there who knows about your pregnancy and understands how to react in an emergency.

14. **Exit the Pool Safely:** When leaving the pool, utilize pool stairs or a ramp to prevent stressing your abdominal muscles.

Swimming is a safe and effective method to keep active and maintain fitness throughout pregnancy. However, it's crucial to be attentive to your comfort and well-being. If you have any concerns or suffer strange swimming symptoms, speak with your healthcare physician soon. They can guide and ensure that swimming stays a safe and fun part of your pregnancy routine.

Stationary Cycling

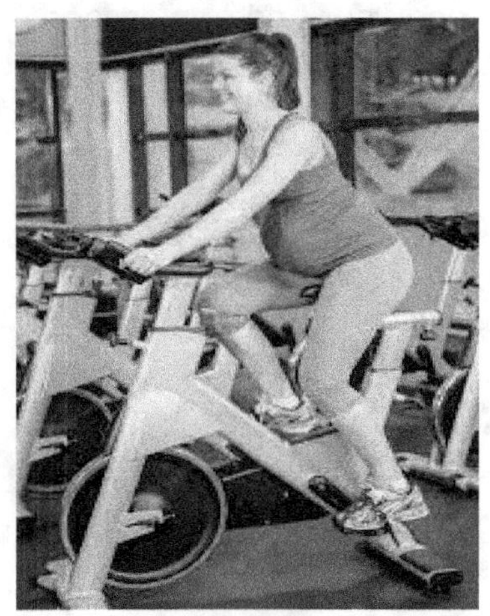

Stationary cycling is a low-impact and safe exercise for pregnant women that gives cardiovascular benefits while reducing joint stress. It's a beautiful approach to maintaining fitness, enhancing energy levels, and promoting general health throughout pregnancy. Here are some advice and instructions for stationary cycling during pregnancy:

1. Speak to Your Healthcare practitioner: Before beginning or maintaining a stationary cycling regimen during pregnancy, speak with your healthcare practitioner. They may analyze your health and pregnancy status and advise based on your circumstances.

2. Use a Stationary Bike: Choose a stationary bike or workout bike with a comfortable seat and customizable settings. Ensure that the bike is in excellent operational condition.

3. Adjust the Seat Height: Adjust the seat height to a level, allowing for a modest knee bend while your foot is near the bottom of the pedal stroke. This posture helps avoid strain on the knees.

4. Maintain a Good stance: While riding, maintain an upright stance with your back straight and shoulders relaxed. Engage your core muscles softly to support your lower back.

5. Warm-Up: Start with a gradual warm-up by pedaling slowly and comfortably for 5-10 minutes. This helps prepare your muscles and joints for the activity.

6. Control the Resistance: Adjust the resistance level to a comfortable setting. Avoid excessive amounts of resistance that might strain your muscles or joints.

7. Keep hydrated: Drink water before, during, and after your stationary cycling activity to keep well-hydrated.

8. Monitor Your Heart Rate: Aim to maintain your heart rate within a reasonable range. You should be able to chat comfortably while riding without getting unduly breathless.

9. Listen to Your Body: Heed your body's messages. Slow down or stop immediately if you encounter any pain, dizziness, shortness of breath, or discomfort.

10. Use Pedal Straps: If the bike has pedal straps, use these to keep your feet secure when pedaling.

11. Cool Down: After your exercise, cool down by cycling at a moderate and easy speed for 5-10 minutes. This helps gradually reduce your heart rate.

12. Stretch: Incorporate easy stretching activities to enhance flexibility and minimize muscular tension after your bike workout.

13. Avoid High-Impact Movements: Stationary cycling is preferred to outdoor riding during pregnancy because it avoids the danger of falls or accidents associated with road cycling.

14. Keep Track of Time: Limit your stationary cycling workouts to a comfortable time, generally 20-30 minutes, depending on your fitness level and feelings.

Stationary cycling may be a safe and efficient technique to maintain cardiovascular fitness throughout pregnancy. However, it's crucial to prioritize your comfort and safety. Suppose you have any concerns or suffer strange symptoms while cycling, check with your healthcare physician soon. They can guide and ensure that stationary cycling stays a safe and pleasurable part of your pregnancy regimen.

Low-Impact Aerobics

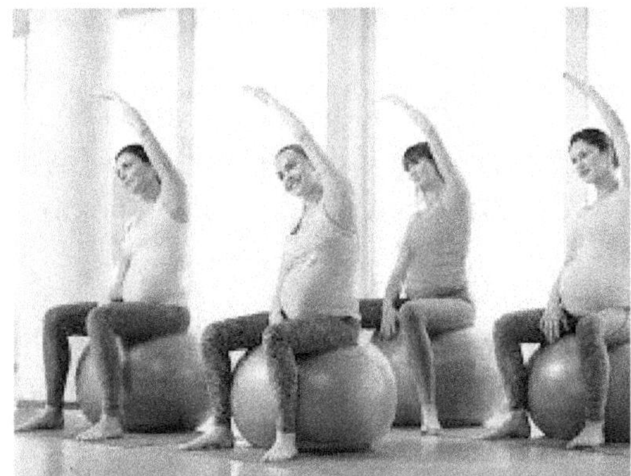

Low-impact aerobics is a terrific alternative for pregnant women wanting to keep active and maintain cardiovascular fitness without putting undue pressure on their joints and ligaments. It incorporates aerobic movements that limit high-impact or jarring actions, making it a safe and effective exercise alternative during pregnancy. Here are some ideas and instructions for low-impact aerobics during pregnancy:

1. Speak to Your Healthcare physician: Before beginning or maintaining a low-impact aerobics regimen during pregnancy, speak with your physician. They may analyze your health and pregnancy status and advise based on your circumstances.

2. Choose a Qualified Instructor: Join a prenatal aerobics class or work with an instructor competent in teaching fitness routines tailored to pregnant women. This ensures that the activities are safe and suitable for your stage of pregnancy.

3. Wear Supportive Footwear: Wear supportive and comfortable sporting shoes with adequate padding to enhance stability and lessen foot and leg pain risk.

4. Dress Comfortably: Wear loose-fitting, breathable clothes that allow for flexibility of movement. Layer garments as required to adjust to changing weather conditions.

5. Warm-Up: Start with a simple warm-up to prepare your muscles and joints for the activity. Perform gentle stretching and deep breathing exercises.

6. Maintain excellent Posture: Throughout the exercise, maintain excellent posture. Stand or move with straight back shoulders relaxed, and use your core muscles lightly.

7. Control Intensity: Control the intensity of your motions and workouts. Avoid leaping or rapid movements that might strain your muscles or joints.

8. Alter as Needed: Be prepared to alter workouts as your pregnancy advances. Some motions may become painful or difficult to execute as you proceed through successive trimesters.

9. Be hydrated: Drink water before, during, and after your low-impact aerobics workout to be well-hydrated.

10. Listen to Your Body: Heed your body's messages. Slow down or stop immediately if you encounter any pain, dizziness, shortness of breath, or discomfort.

11. Cool Down: After your workout, cool down with easy stretching activities to enhance flexibility and minimize muscular tension.

12. Breathing: Focus on regulated and rhythmic breathing throughout the exercises. Inhale deeply through your nose and exhale slowly through your mouth.

13. Regular Attendance: Attend low-impact aerobics sessions frequently since consistency is critical for maintaining fitness throughout pregnancy.

Low-impact aerobics may help pregnant women keep active, enhance cardiovascular health, and raise energy levels. It may also give social support and a feeling of community while attending lessons with other pregnant women. However, it's vital to prioritize your comfort and safety. If you have any concerns or suffer strange symptoms during your exercise, check with your healthcare physician soon. They may give direction and guarantee that low-impact aerobics stays a safe and pleasant part of your pregnancy regimen.

Elliptical Trainer

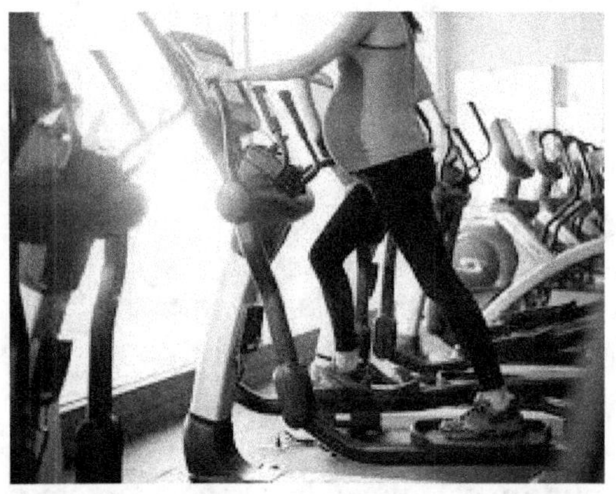

Using an elliptical trainer is a low-impact and safe exercise for pregnant women that gives cardiovascular benefits while reducing joint stress. It's a beautiful approach to maintain fitness, enhance endurance, and boosting general health throughout pregnancy. Here are some suggestions and instructions for utilizing an elliptical trainer during pregnancy:

1. Speak with Your Healthcare practitioner: Before beginning or maintaining an elliptical trainer regimen during pregnancy, speak with your healthcare practitioner. They may analyze your health and pregnancy status and advise based on your circumstances.

2. Choose a Safe Elliptical Machine: Use a high-quality elliptical trainer with customizable settings. Ensure that the machine is in excellent functioning condition.

3. Adjust the Resistance: Start with a modest resistance level and progressively raise it as your fitness level permits. Avoid excessive amounts of resistance that might strain your muscles or joints.

4. Maintain Good Posture: While utilizing the elliptical machine, stand up straight with your back aligned and Shoulders relaxed. Engage your core muscles softly to support your lower back.

5. Warm-Up: Start with a gradual warm-up by utilizing the elliptical slowly and comfortably for 5-10 minutes. This helps prepare your muscles and joints for the activity.

6. Keep hydrated: Drink water before, during, and after your elliptical activity to keep well-hydrated.

7. Control Your Heart Rate: Aim to maintain your heart rate within a reasonable range. You should be able to chat comfortably while using the elliptical without getting unduly breathless.

8. Listen to Your Body: Heed your body's messages. Slow down or stop immediately if you encounter any pain, dizziness, shortness of breath, or discomfort.

9. Use Handlebars Safely: If the elliptical trainer has handlebars, use them for stability and balance. Avoid excessive twisting or spinning motions with the handlebars.

10. Cool Down: After your exercise, cool down by riding the elliptical at a moderate and easy speed for 5-10 minutes. This helps gradually reduce your heart rate.

11. Stretch: Incorporate mild stretching activities to increase flexibility and alleviate muscular tension after your elliptical activity.

12. Avoid Overheating: Be conscious of your body temperature. Use a fan or guarantee appropriate ventilation if using an elliptical at home.

13. Regular Exercise: Add elliptical training sessions consistently in your fitness plan since consistency is crucial to maintaining cardiovascular fitness throughout pregnancy.

14. Change as Needed: As your pregnancy advances, you may need to change your elliptical regimen or lessen the time of your exercises. Be adaptable and alter your exercises to fit your changing demands.

Elliptical training is a safe and efficient strategy to keep active and maintain cardiovascular fitness throughout pregnancy. However, it's crucial to prioritize your comfort and safety. If you have any concerns or suffer strange symptoms while using the elliptical trainer, check with your healthcare physician soon. They may give direction and ensure that elliptical exercising stays a safe and fun component of your pregnancy regimen.

Dancing

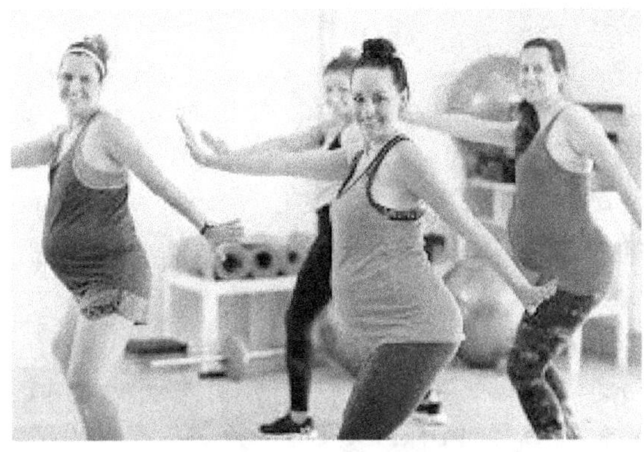

Dancing may be a pleasant and engaging exercise for pregnant women, providing it is done correctly and with specific adaptations to meet the changes in your body during pregnancy. Here are some advice and rules for dancing during pregnancy:

1. Speak with Your Healthcare physician: Before beginning or maintaining a dance regimen during pregnancy, speak with your physician. They may analyze your health and pregnancy status and advise based on your circumstances.

2. Choose Suitable Dance types: Opt for low-impact dance types that are easy on the joints. Styles including prenatal dance, ballet, lyrical, and various kinds of contemporary dance might be suited. Avoid high-impact dances, especially ones that include leaping and forceful motions.

3. Take Prenatal Dance courses: Look for prenatal dance courses offered by teachers with expertise in dealing with pregnant mothers. These sessions are meant to give pregnant women safe and acceptable dancing routines.

4. Adapt moves: Be prepared to adapt dancing moves to meet your changing physique. As your pregnancy advances, you may need to reduce or remove specific steps or leaps to minimize strain.

5. Wear Supportive Footwear: Choose comfortable and supportive dancing shoes with appropriate cushioning and stability to reduce foot and leg strain.

6. Dress Comfortably: Wear loose-fitting, breathable clothes that allow for flexibility of movement. Layer garments as required to adjust to changing weather conditions.

7. Warm-Up and Cool Down: Start each dancing practice with a simple warm-up, which may involve stretching and light movements. Finish with a cool-down phase to gradually drop your heart rate and rest your muscles.

8. Maintain proper Posture: While dancing, maintain proper posture. Stand or move with your back aligned and shoulders relaxed. Engage your core muscles softly to support your lower back.

9. Listen to Your Body: Heed your body's messages. If you encounter any pain, dizziness, shortness of breath, or discomfort, pause and relax.

10. Be Hydrated: Drink water before, during, and after your dancing session to be well-hydrated.

11. Avoid Overheating: Be careful of your body temperature. Ensure appropriate ventilation and consider dancing in a well-ventilated location.

12. Choose Suitable Music: Select music with a reasonable pace that enables you to dance easily without overexertion.

13. Use Props Sparingly: If you add props or accessories to your dancing performance, use them sparingly and carefully to prevent mishaps or strain.

14. Social Dancing: If you like social dancing, such as ballroom or salsa, continue participating, but be careful of abrupt or violent moves that may impact your balance.

15. Partner Dancing: In partner dances, talk with your dance partner about your pregnancy and any required changes to moves.

16. Regular Practice: Try to dance often to maintain fitness and enjoy the emotional advantages of dancing.

However, alter your regimen as required to fit your shifting demands and energy levels.

Dancing during pregnancy may be pleasurable and gratifying to keep active and maintain your health. However, it's crucial to prioritize your comfort and safety, make any adaptations, and communicate with your healthcare physician if you have any concerns or encounter unexpected symptoms. With the correct safeguards, you may continue to enjoy dancing as a part of your pregnancy routine.

CHAPTER FIVE

Strength Training for a Healthy Pregnancy

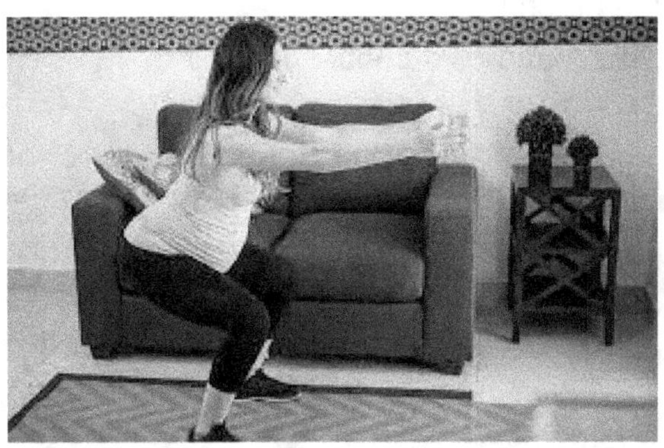

Strength training is a critical component of a healthy pregnancy, as it may help increase muscle tone, promote improved posture, and prepare your body for the physical demands of labor and birthing. Here are five strength training activities that are typically safe for pregnant women, but it's vital to contact your healthcare professional before beginning any new fitness regimen, particularly during pregnancy:

1. **Squats:**
   - Stand with your feet hip-width apart.
   - Engage your core muscles.
   - Lower your body by bending your knees and hips as if sitting back in a chair.
   - Keep your back straight and chest raised.
   - Aim to drop until your thighs are parallel to the ground or at a comfortable depth.
   - Push through your heels to return to the starting position.

- Perform 2-3 sets of 10-15 repetitions.

2. **Seated Rows:**
   - Sit on a stable chair or bench with your back straight and feet level on the ground.
   - Hold a resistance band or dumbbell in front of you with your arms outstretched.
   - Bend your elbows, bringing the resistance band or weights toward your body.
   - Squeeze your shoulder blades together while you do this.
   - Slowly relax and straighten your arms.
   - Perform 2-3 sets of 10-15 repetitions.

3. **Push-Ups (Modified):**
   - Begin in a kneeling posture with your hands on the floor shoulder-width apart.
   - Keep your back straight and your core engaged.
   - Lower your chest towards the ground by bending your elbows.
   - Push back up to the starting position.
   - You may also practice wall push-ups or use an incline to simplify this workout.
   - Perform 2-3 sets of 8-12 repetitions.

4. **Planks:**
   - Start in a hands-and-knee posture with your wrists precisely beneath your shoulders.
   - Extend your legs behind you, maintaining your body in a straight line.

- Engage your core muscles and maintain this posture for as long as comfortable, aiming for 20-30 seconds initially and progressively increasing the duration as your strength develops.
- Make sure not to arch your back or allow your hips to sag.

5. **Bicep Curls:**
   - Hold a dumbbell in each hand, with your arms outstretched at your sides and palms facing front.
   - Keep your back straight and core engaged.
   - Bend your elbows, raising the weights towards your shoulders.
   - Lower the weights back to the starting position.
   - Perform 2-3 sets of 10-15 repetitions.

Remember to employ good form and technique for each exercise, and start with modest weights or resistance bands if you're new to strength training. Gradually increase the weight or resistance as your strength develops. Listen to your body; if any activity produces discomfort or pain, quit it and talk with your healthcare professional. Additionally, it's vital to warm up before strength training and to conduct stretching exercises to enhance flexibility and minimize muscular tension after your workout.

CHAPTER SIX

Pelvic Floor and Core Strengthening

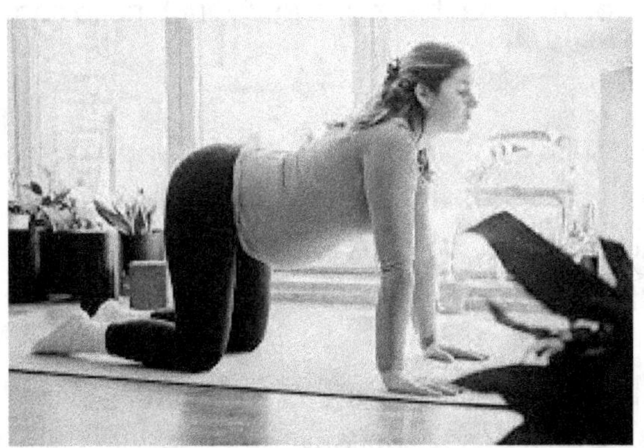

Pelvic floor and core strengthening exercises are crucial throughout pregnancy and after to assist your body as it experiences considerable changes. Strong pelvic floor and core muscles help avoid concerns like incontinence and stabilize your developing tummy. Here are some safe and efficient exercises for pelvic floor and core strengthening during pregnancy:

1. Kegel Exercises:
- Kegel exercises target the pelvic floor muscles, vital for bladder control and supporting the uterus.
- To execute a Kegel exercise, consider attempting to halt the flow of pee midstream. Contract the muscles you use for this activity without activating your abdominal, buttock, or thigh muscles.
- Hold the contraction for 5-10 seconds, then relax simultaneously.

- Repeat this exercise 10-15 times in a row, many times a day.

2. Pelvic Tilts:

- Pelvic tilts assist in strengthening your lower back and core muscles.
- Start on your hands and knees with a neutral spine (back flat).
- Inhale and exhale as you circle your back, tucking your pelvis under (like a cat stretching).
- Inhale again and return to a neutral spine.
- Perform 10-15 repetitions.

3. Modified Planks:

- Planks may help strengthen your core, but the reduced form is safer during pregnancy.
- Begin in a hands-and-knee posture.
- Lower onto your forearms and stretch your legs behind you, maintaining your body in a straight line from head to heels.
- Hold this posture for as long as comfortable, aiming for 20-30 seconds initially and then increasing the duration as your strength develops.
- Make sure not to arch your back or allow your hips to sag.

4. Seated Leg Lifts:

- Sit on a chair or the edge of a bench with your back straight and feet flat on the floor.
- Hold onto the edges of the chair for support.

- Lift one foot a few inches off the ground, keeping your knee bent at a 90-degree angle.
- Lower your foot back to the ground and repeat with the opposite leg.
- Perform 10-15 reps on each leg.

5. Pelvic Clocks:
- Pelvic clocks assist in raising awareness of your pelvic posture and develop the deep core muscles.
- Sit or lay down with your knees bent and feet flat on the floor.
- Imagine your pelvis as the face of a clock.
- Tilt your pelvis forward (noon), to the right (3 o'clock), back (6 o'clock), and then to the left (9 o'clock) in a calm and controlled way.
- Perform 10-15 repetitions in each direction.

Always emphasize good form and technique throughout these workouts. If you suffer pain, discomfort, or odd sensations while completing these exercises, stop immediately and talk with your healthcare physician. They can recommend the most effective workouts for your unique requirements and stage of pregnancy.

CHAPTER SEVEN

Managing Pregnancy Aches and Pains

Relieving Back Pain

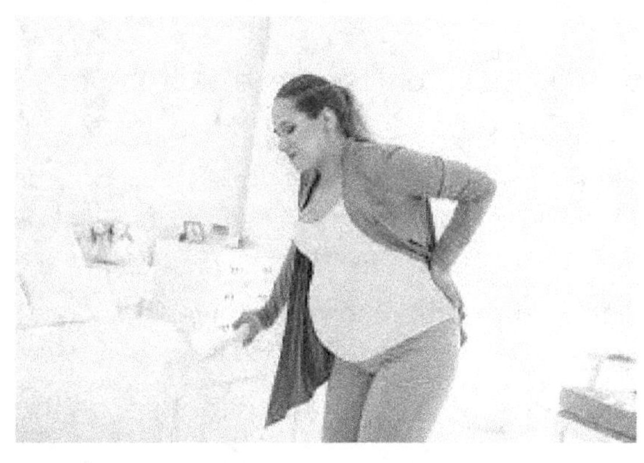

Back pain is a frequent issue during pregnancy due to the changes in your body's posture and the extra weight of the developing baby. While it's vital to speak with your healthcare professional for individualized guidance, here are some basic suggestions and exercises that may help reduce back discomfort during pregnancy:

1. Maintain Good Posture:
- Stand up straight with your shoulders back.
- Use a cushion or lumbar roll to support the natural curvature of your lower back while sitting.
- When lifting something, bend at the knees and utilize your leg muscles rather than your back.

2. Gentle Stretches:

- **Cat-Cow Stretch:** On your hands and knees, arch your back upward (cat) and then arch it downward (cow). Repeat this action slowly.
- **Child's Pose:** Kneel on the floor with your big toes touching and knees apart. Sit back into your heels and stretch your arms forward, lowering your chest towards the ground.
- **Hip Flexor Stretch:** Kneel on one knee with the other foot in front and slowly bend forward. Hold for 20-30 seconds and swap sides.

3. Pelvic Tilt Exercises:

- Pelvic tilts assist in strengthening your lower back and abdominal muscles.
- Lie on your back with your legs bent and feet flat on the floor.
- Tighten your abdominal muscles and push your lower back against the floor. Hold for a few seconds, then release.
- Perform 10-15 repetitions.

4. Prenatal Yoga & Pilates:

- Prenatal yoga and Pilates programs may give gentle stretches and strengthening exercises geared to pregnancy. Look for lessons conducted by qualified teachers.

5. Heat and Cold Therapy:

- Applying a warm compress or warm bath might help relax tense muscles.
- Cold packs may decrease inflammation and give comfort when applied to the affected region.

6. Supportive Footwear:

- Wear comfortable and supportive shoes that might help prevent back discomfort, mainly if your feet swell during pregnancy.

7. Prenatal Massage:

- Consider having a prenatal massage from a skilled therapist specializing in pregnant massage. They might target areas of stress and pain.

8. Prenatal Exercise:

- Regular, mild exercise may help strengthen your core and back muscles, improving posture and lowering back discomfort. Consult your healthcare physician for proper workout advice.

9. Sleep Support:

- Use a body or a pregnant pillow to support your body while sleeping. Sleeping on your side with a cushion between your knees might also reduce back aches.

10. Consult a Chiropractor or Physical Therapist:

- Some pregnant women find relief via chiropractic treatment or physical therapy. Ensure you find a practitioner skilled in dealing with pregnant patients.

Remember that it's vital to contact your healthcare physician before attempting any new activities or therapies to verify they are safe and suitable for your unique situation. If you suffer severe or chronic back pain, unexpected discomfort changes, or other concerns, call your healthcare professional quickly for examination and counseling.

Dealing with Swelling and Discomfort

Swelling and pain, particularly in the legs and feet, are prevalent during pregnancy due to increased blood volume, hormonal changes, and the pressure of the expanding uterus on blood vessels. While it's vital to speak with your healthcare professional for individualized guidance, here are some basic techniques and methods to assist in decreasing swelling and pain during pregnancy:

1. Rest and Elevate:

- Elevating your legs whenever feasible might help minimize edema. Prop your legs up on pillows or a cushion when relaxing or sleeping.
- Avoid sitting or standing for lengthy durations. Take brief pauses to lift your legs and alter positions.

2. Compression Stockings:

- Graduated compression stockings may assist in increasing blood circulation and minimize edema. Consult your healthcare physician for guidance on the correct degree of compression and suitable size.

3. Stay Hydrated:

- Drink lots of water to help remove extra fluids from your body. Staying hydrated may also help avoid constipation, which can lead to pain.

4. Watch Your Salt Intake:

- Excessive salt (sodium) may lead to fluid retention. Reduce your sodium consumption by avoiding highly processed and salty meals.

5. Gentle Exercise:

- Engaging in low-impact workouts like walking, swimming, or prenatal yoga may improve circulation and minimize edema.

6. Avoid Tight Clothing:

- Wear loose-fitting, comfortable clothes to allow for greater blood flow. Avoid tight waistbands and socks with tight elastic tops.

7. Massage:

- Gently massage your legs, ankles, and feet to increase circulation and alleviate stress. Use upward strokes toward the heart.

8. Cool Compresses:
- Applying a cold compress to inflamed regions might help decrease inflammation and give comfort. Use a towel soaked in cold water or an excellent gel pack.

9. Avoid Crossing Your Legs:
- Crossing your legs might hinder blood flow. Try to sit flat on the ground or a footrest.

10. Foot Exercises: - Ankle circles and toe flexes might assist in improving circulation in your feet. Perform these exercises frequently throughout the day.

11. Supportive Footwear: - Wear comfortable shoes with solid arch support to ease pain and lower the risk of foot edema.

12. Pregnancy cushion: - A pregnancy cushion may support and ease pain while sleeping. Use it to support your legs, hips, and back as required.

13. Talk to Your Healthcare Provider: - If swelling is severe, abrupt, or accompanied by other troubling symptoms (such as elevated blood pressure or headaches), visit your healthcare practitioner soon, as it might indicate a more severe problem.

14. Consider Alternative treatments: - Some pregnant women find comfort via treatments such as acupuncture, acupressure, or reflexology. Ensure you find a practitioner skilled in dealing with pregnant people.

Remember that although modest swelling is usual during pregnancy, monitoring it and discussing any concerns with your healthcare professional is vital. They may analyze your situation, rule out any underlying concerns, and give specific counsel to help manage your pain and swelling successfully.

Modifications for Common Issues

Pregnancy may bring about many discomforts and problems, but there are typically adaptations and methods that can help reduce these concerns. Here are some frequent pregnancy concerns and possible modifications:

1. Morning Sickness:
- Eat small, frequent meals throughout the day to avoid an empty stomach.
- Avoid hot, oily, and strong-smelling meals that might provoke nausea.
- Stay hydrated by consuming water or ginger tea.

2. Fatigue:
- Prioritize relaxation and sleep. Take brief naps throughout the day if required.
- Delegate chores and responsibilities to lessen physical and mental strain.
- Modify your workout program to incorporate milder kinds of movement, like pregnant yoga.

3. Heartburn:

- Eat smaller meals to prevent overfilling your tummy.
- Avoid lying down shortly after eating. Stay upright for at least 2-3 hours.
- Choose items that are less prone to provoke heartburn, such as plain yogurt and oats.

4. Back Pain:

- Maintain proper posture by standing up straight and utilizing supportive seats.
- Perform mild stretches and exercises to improve your core and back muscles.
- Use a pregnant pillow to support your body while sleeping.

5. Swelling and Discomfort:

- Elevate your legs while resting to decrease edema.
- Wear comfortable, loose-fitting clothes and supportive footwear.
- Engage in mild activity like walking to enhance circulation.

6. Shortness of Breath:

- Practice deep breathing techniques to enhance lung capacity and lessen anxiety.
- Modify your workout plan to incorporate lower-intensity activities like swimming.
- Avoid severe physical activity.

7. Constipation:

- Increase your fiber intake by eating more fruits, veggies, and whole grains.
- Stay hydrated by drinking lots of water throughout the day.
- Engage in frequent, mild exercise to support healthy bowel motions.

8. Pelvic Pain and Discomfort:

- Use a pregnancy support belt or band to offer extra support to your pelvis.
- Avoid standing for extended periods and take pauses to sit or lay down.
- Perform modest pelvic tilts and stretches to reduce pain.

9. Leg Cramps:

- Stay hydrated and ensure you receive adequate calcium and magnesium in your diet.
- Stretch your legs before night and gently massage your calf muscles.
- Sleep with your feet raised on a pillow.

10. Varicose Veins:

- Wear compression stockings to promote blood circulation.
- Elevate your legs while resting to decrease strain on the veins.
- Engage in frequent, low-impact exercise to promote general circulation.

-

11. Round Ligament Pain:
- Use mild stretches to reduce stress in the abdominal region.
- Avoid unexpected movements or postures that generate acute discomfort.
- Apply a warm compress to the afflicted region for relief.

12. Hormonal Changes and Emotional Health:
- Practice relaxation methods such as deep breathing, meditation, or prenatal yoga.
- Seek emotional support from friends, family, or a counselor if required.
- Prioritize self-care and indulge in things that offer you pleasure and relaxation.

Remember that every pregnancy is unique; what works for one person may not work for another. It's crucial to discuss with your healthcare practitioner about any concerns or pain you are experiencing. They may give tailored assistance, propose necessary alterations, and address any concerns you may have to promote a safe and pleasant pregnancy.

CHAPTER EIGHT

Nutrition and Hydration During Pregnancy

Importance of Proper Nutrition

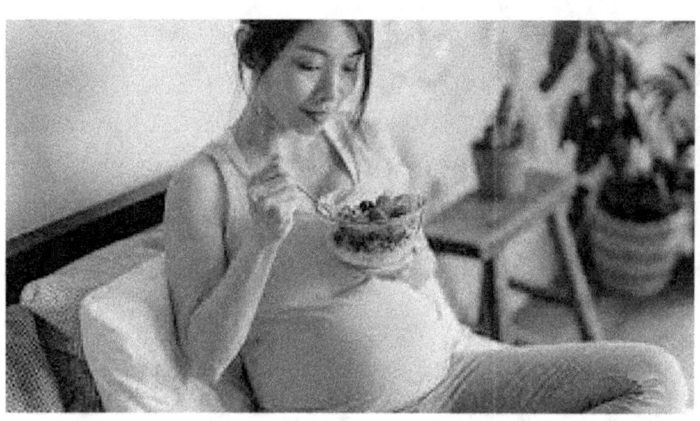

Proper nutrition throughout pregnancy is vital for both the expecting woman's health and the developing baby's growth. It is vital in supporting several aspects of pregnancy, including the mother's health, fetal development, and general well-being. Here are the primary reasons why a healthy diet is vital for pregnant women:

1. Fetal Development:
- Adequate nutrition supplies essential nutrients, including folic acid, iron, calcium, and numerous vitamins necessary for developing the baby's brain, spinal cord, organs, and bones.

2. Preventing Birth Defects:
- Proper nutrition, notably the consumption of folic acid before and throughout early pregnancy, may dramatically

lower the incidence of neural tube abnormalities, such as spina bifida.

3. Maternal Health:
- A well-balanced diet helps the health of the expecting woman by helping to avoid issues including anemia, gestational diabetes, and preeclampsia.

4. Energy and Stamina:
- Pregnancy exerts higher physical demands on the body. An adequate diet offers the energy and stamina required to deal with various demands, including weight increase and changes in body composition.

5. Healthy Weight Gain:
- Gaining an adequate amount of weight during pregnancy is vital for the health of both the mother and baby. Proper eating helps control weight growth and prevent the danger of excessive or insufficient weight gain.

6. Blood Volume Increase:

- Pregnancy leads to an increase in blood volume to support the developing fetus. Proper nutrition, especially iron-rich meals, helps prevent anemia and provides sufficient oxygen flow to the mother and fetus.

7. Immune System Support:
- A balanced diet helps maintain the immune system, minimizing the risk of infections and sickness during pregnancy, which may harm the baby.

8. Hormonal Balance:

- Hormonal changes during pregnancy might impact appetite and digestion. A balanced diet helps maintain hormonal balance and manage pregnancy-related symptoms, including nausea and constipation.

9. Bone Health:

- Calcium and vitamin D consumption is crucial for supporting the mother's and newborn's bone health. A proper diet improves the development of the baby's bones and helps avoid maternal bone loss.

10. Lactation and Postpartum Recovery:

- A well-nourished woman is better equipped for nursing, as she will have the required nutrients to assist milk production and recovery after delivery.

11. Psychological Well-being:

- A proper diet may significantly benefit pregnant women's mental and emotional well-being, lowering the risk of mood disorders, including depression.

12. Long-Term Health:

- Proper nutrition during pregnancy may impact the baby's health, lowering the chance of chronic illnesses like obesity and diabetes later in life.

To ensure optimal nutrition throughout pregnancy, pregnant moms must maintain a balanced and varied diet, contact a healthcare practitioner for nutritional counseling, and take prenatal vitamins as advised. A licensed dietitian or nutritionist with experience in prenatal nutrition may also give vital guidance to promote a healthy pregnancy. Proper nutrition is a crucial component of prenatal care and is significant in promoting a healthy pregnancy and a flourishing infant.

Hydration Tips for Active Moms-to-Be

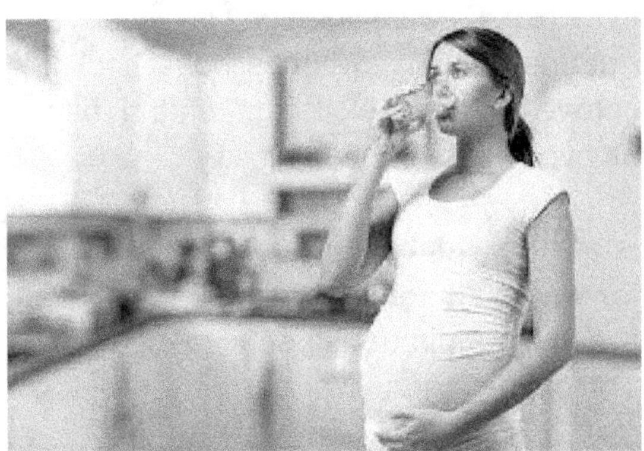

Staying well-hydrated is vital for all pregnant women, particularly active ones who participate in frequent exercise. Proper hydration maintains general health, helps avoid difficulties, and protects the well-being of the expecting woman and the developing infant. Here are some hydration strategies for active moms-to-be:

1. Drink Water Throughout the Day:
- Sip water consistently throughout the day rather than waiting until you're thirsty. This helps maintain a steady amount of hydration.

2. Monitor Urine Color:
- Pay attention to the color of your pee. Pale, light yellow pee indicates healthy hydration, but dark yellow or amber urine may suggest dehydration.

3. Pre-Hydrate Before Exercise:
- Drink water before commencing your workout program to ensure you are fully hydrated.

4. Stay Hydrated During Exercise:
- While exercising, take frequent water breaks to keep hydrated. Sip modest amounts of water rather than ingesting significant volumes simultaneously to prevent discomfort.

5. Rehydrate After Exercise:
- After exercise, rehydrate by consuming water to replenish fluids lost via sweat.

6. Consider Sports Drinks Sparingly:
- While water is usually the best option for hydration, sports beverages containing electrolytes may be helpful for longer, more strenuous exercises. However, use them cautiously and speak with your healthcare practitioner for suggestions.

7. Monitor Weather Conditions:
- Be careful of hot and humid conditions, as you may need to increase your fluid intake to account for increased perspiration.

8. Listen to Your Body:
- Pay heed to your body's messages. If you feel thirsty, drink water. Thirst is a natural signal that your body needs water.

9. Include Hydrating Foods:

- Incorporate hydrating items into your diet, such as water-rich fruits (e.g., watermelon, oranges) and vegetables (e.g., cucumber, celery).

10. Limit Caffeine and Sugary Drinks:

- Limit your consumption of caffeinated beverages and sugary drinks since these may lead to dehydration. Water is the most excellent option for hydration during pregnancy.

11. Be Mindful of Signs of Dehydration:

- Watch for indicators of dehydration, including dark urine, dry mouth, dizziness, fast pulse, and decreased urine production. If you have any of these symptoms, increase your fluid intake.

12. Consult Your Healthcare Practitioner:

- Discuss your exercise regimen and hydration requirements with your healthcare practitioner. They may make customized advice depending on your circumstances and exercise level.

13. Adjust Hydration for Intensity and Duration:

- The intensity and length of your exercises will alter your hydration demands. Longer or more strenuous exercises may necessitate more hydration consumption.

14. Plan for Hydration During Activities:
- If you're engaged in activities away from home, plan by having a reusable water bottle.

15. Hydrate for Recovery:
- Emphasize water for recovery after exercise. This helps your body replace fluids, aids muscular recovery, and minimizes the chance of cramping.

Remember that every pregnancy is unique, and water requirements might vary. It's vital to check with your healthcare professional for individualized information on remaining well-hydrated while maintaining an active lifestyle throughout pregnancy. Proper hydration is vital for your and your kid's health and well-being.